EAT TO HEAL

The ASTR Diet: Unlock the Healing Power of Food to End Sickness and Thrive

ASTR

Second Edition

Official ASTR Diet Book

Dr. Joseph Jacobs, DPT, ACN

Second Edition, January 2026

Published by ASTR Institute
614 E HWY 50 #169, Clermont, FL 34711

ASTRinstitute.com

ASTR

Disclaimer

This book, authored by Dr. Joseph Jacobs and published by the ASTR Institute, is intended for informational purposes only and presents medical research findings. It is not a substitute for professional medical advice, diagnosis, or treatment. Dr. Joseph Jacobs, the ASTR Institute, and its affiliates do not endorse or assume responsibility for any specific medical treatments or procedures discussed in this book. We strongly advise readers to consult with their healthcare providers regarding the applicability of any aspects of the content to their own health and well-being.

The statements contained herein have not been evaluated by the Food and Drug Administration. The products mentioned are not designed to diagnose, cure, treat, or prevent any disease. Individual results may vary, and we cannot guarantee that you will achieve the same outcomes as those detailed in our case studies, testimonials, and treatment videos. Success varies per individual, and one person's results do not guarantee similar outcomes for another.

If you have medical concerns, consult with your healthcare provider, physician, or another qualified medical professional. Dr. Joseph Jacobs, the ASTR Institute, and their associated organizations and individuals disclaim any liability for actions, services, or products acquired through this book, our videos, website, or any of our media channels.

Table of Contents

Dedication

To my wife,

Thank you for your constant support and encouragement throughout my journey with chronic pain. Your love and belief in me have been invaluable, especially as I worked on my inventions and pursued solutions to help others. This book would not have been possible without you by my side.

Eat to Heal: A Guide to the ASTR Diet is also lovingly dedicated to my children as part of their homeschool curriculum, instilling in them the knowledge and importance of nutrition for lifelong health. It is dedicated to my patients as well, with the hope of empowering them to take charge of their health by understanding how to use food as medicine. This book serves as a tool to inspire individuals to harness the healing power of nutrition, supporting their journey toward a healthier, more vibrant life.

Triumph Over Trials

Triumph Over Trials

After my second cancer treatment, I was suffering from chronic fatigue, migraines, muscle and joint pain. I reached out to at least seven doctors, but I could not find relief. Unfortunately, they had two responses. First, they said my blood labs looked normal. I learned from my studies in nutrition that this happened because they did not order the correct labs to figure out the root cause of my issues. The second response was that I was a hopeless case. This made me realize that if I wanted to overcome my disability, I had to look for a solution on my own. It was a difficult time in my life. Due to my pain and fatigue, it used to take me 10 minutes just to walk from the living room to the bathroom, about 20 feet away. I was very depressed and angry because, at 30 years old, I was facing numerous health issues and had a poor quality of life without any answers.

I spent countless hours and years studying nutrition, psychology, behavioral modification, anatomy, physiology, ergonomics, and other medical topics in hopes of finding an answer. At the same time, I was frustrated that the techniques I learned in medical school only provided short-term results with no lasting relief. I tried what I learned in school, such as stretching, exercises, electrical stimulation, various massage techniques, manual therapy, joint mobilization, and myofascial release, but nothing provided long-term results. So, I started to look at medical studies to guide me through this process. After reviewing over 16,000 medical research papers with assistance from medical students, I was shocked and disappointed by the results. Based on these studies, the following treatments either provided no pain reduction or only short-term pain reduction:

- NSAIDs
- Opioids
- Cortisone shots
- Exercises
- Stretching
- Massage
- Joint mobilization or manipulation
- Acupuncture

- Dry needling
- Instrument-assisted soft tissue mobilization

I have dedicated my life to researching all current traditional medical approaches to treating pain. I've found that the majority of these approaches primarily focus on relieving symptoms rather than addressing the root cause of the pain. The techniques I learned in school, still used in today's modern medical world, have their origins in ancient healing practices such as manipulation, massage, stretching, and exercise. These methods were used by the Romans, Greeks, and Egyptians to increase flexibility, strengthen muscles, and alleviate pain. Today's medicine has added treatments like cold, heat, electrical stimulation, and joint adjustment to this list. However, overwhelming evidence from published medical studies shows no promising long-term relief from any of these methods.

For instance, one systematic review conducted by the University of Ottawa, Canada, which reviewed 270 research studies, concluded that the benefits of massage, acupuncture, and spine adjustment treatments were mostly evident immediately or shortly after treatment, then faded over time. With compelling data like this, it is perplexing how we continue to treat patients with modalities that do not effectively address their long-term needs. Instead of focusing so much on the body's symptoms, we need to start questioning why these symptoms are present in the first place and why they keep returning.

This question guided me through an intense investigative research process over five years. From this research, I concluded that there are seven aspects of chronic pain that, when treated simultaneously, can lead to long-term pain relief. In my book, **Pain No More**, I outline seven key elements that must be addressed simultaneously to effectively relieve chronic pain. I also found that the BioPsychosocial model is an effective treatment approach for long-term pain reduction. So, I studied the BioPsychosocial model in depth and realized that my medical education was lacking in nutrition knowledge. I spent thousands of hours reading and studying nutrition and bought any book that I felt could help me understand the body better.

During this time, my wife had chronic jaw pain due to stress at work. I tried everything I learned from school on her, but nothing provided long-term pain relief. One day she woke up with lockjaw, unable to speak or open her mouth. She asked me to try anything. I told her that I had tried everything I knew, but nothing worked. So, I reached inside her mouth and experimented with several maneuvers. After a few minutes, she was able to open her mouth and was pain-free. I was dumbfounded and had no idea what had just happened. It took me several days to understand the physiology of the maneuvers I had performed. I then started experimenting with the same concept, applying it to the whole body to relieve both my pain and my patients' pain.

After several months of using my hands to implement the new maneuvers I had come up with, I realized I could not do that long-term. My hands were very sore, and I suffered from pain every night. I told my wife that this was not sustainable because I was in so much pain from using my hands. While patients were getting relief, I was suffering. My wife suggested that I use tools instead of my hands. So, I went to a hardware store and bought rubber, plastic, and metal to cut and design tools and devices to replace my hand maneuvers. Thankfully, this provided even faster results for my patients without me feeling soreness from working on them.

I was able to overcome my chronic fatigue and migraines by running comprehensive lab tests. These tests revealed several vitamin, mineral, and hormonal imbalances. Additionally, I overcame my chronic joint and muscle pain through the biopsychosocial (BPS) model and the tools and devices I invented. I also reinvented the biopsychosocial model to be implemented by a single healthcare provider and called it ASTR treatment.

My journey toward developing the ASTR diet was driven by personal challenges and professional insights. I experienced significant frustration with various diets that often left me feeling fatigued and unsatisfied. Through an extensive review of research studies, I also uncovered potential health risks associated with extreme dietary approaches. These experiences inspired me to create the ASTR diet as a healthier, evidence-based alternative.

To develop an effective solution, I carefully examined each ingredient, researched its impact on the body, and evaluated its safety and healing potential. Ingredients that supported the body's natural healing processes and demonstrated anti-inflammatory properties were thoughtfully incorporated into the diet. This methodical approach, built on 15 years of dedicated research, resulted in a balanced and restorative dietary framework. My hope is that this book will serve as a practical guide, empowering you to embrace healthier eating habits. It is designed to help you begin a transformative journey toward healing and well-being, grounded in the belief that food can be our most powerful medicine. In the following chapters, I will provide a foundational understanding of nutrition, explore relevant research, introduce the principles of the ASTR diet, and outline clear, actionable steps to ensure its easy and effective implementation.

The Roadmap to Healing

The ASTR Diet Story

For years, I struggled with feeling unwell after eating and tried numerous trendy diets, including Atkins, keto, carnivore, vegan, and vegetarian. Despite my efforts, none of these approaches offered lasting relief. This frustration led me to study nutrition, where I discovered the importance of moderation and the power of anti-inflammatory ingredients. Extreme diets often overlook the body's essential need for a balanced intake of carbohydrates, fats, and proteins, the three macronutrients critical for overall health. Such imbalance can lead to serious health issues, as I explain in the chapter on trendy diets.

To create an effective solution, I carefully examined each ingredient, researched its impact on the body, and evaluated its safety and healing potential. Ingredients that supported the body's natural healing processes and demonstrated anti-inflammatory properties were thoughtfully incorporated into the diet. This methodical approach, built on 15 years of dedicated research, resulted in a balanced and restorative dietary framework. My goal is for this book to serve as a practical guide, empowering you to adopt healthier eating habits. It is designed to help you embark on a transformative journey toward healing and well-being, rooted in the belief that food is our most powerful medicine.

Imagine a car that runs on gasoline as its primary fuel source. If you were to fill the tank with water instead, the car would break down. The same principle applies to our bodies. Consuming refined carbohydrates, chemicals, and microplastics instead of real, nourishing food can gradually contribute to the development of disease. These health issues often take years to manifest and become diagnosable. By the time symptoms appear, the disease is usually in its advanced stages. This underscores the importance of viewing food as either medicine or poison.

United States is facing a health crisis of staggering proportions. Over 73% of Americans are overweight, a chronic condition linked to malnutrition and poor dietary habits. As a doctor, cancer survivor, and advocate for nutrition, I've seen firsthand the damage inflicted by modern diets. To address the root causes of these issues, not just the symptoms, I developed the ASTR Diet (Anti-inflammatory, Sustainable, Toxin-free, Restorative) as a holistic approach to health and well-being.

The ASTR Diet is more than just a meal plan; it's a framework for a healthier, more balanced life built on **15 years of evidence-based research and real-world testing**. This approach was developed through a deep review of nutritional science and clinical studies, combined with hands-on personal evaluation of the most popular diets to identify what truly supports healing and what silently fuels inflammation. By prioritizing anti-inflammatory foods, eliminating toxins, and supporting the body's natural healing processes, the ASTR Diet empowers individuals to take control of their health with a strategy grounded in both science and experience. Whether you're battling chronic pain, fatigue, or simply looking to feel your best, this approach serves as a roadmap to lasting wellness. I hope this book inspires readers to see food as a powerful tool for nourishment and healing, while also recognizing its potential to contribute to illness. My goal is to emphasize the profound impact food choices have on overall health. Through this book, you will learn that food is either poison or medicine.

My aim is for this book to act as a practical resource, enabling you to embrace healthier eating habits. In the following chapters, we explore the hidden toxins we unknowingly consume daily and their profound effects on our health. I will then discuss the foundation of the ASTR diet.

What the ASTR Diet Means

Each component of the ASTR Diet reflects a deliberate choice to prioritize health:

A - Anti-inflammatory: Chronic inflammation is the root cause of many diseases. This diet focuses on foods that calm the body's inflammatory response.

S -Sustainable: A healthy diet must be practical and easy to maintain over the long term.

T - Toxin-free: Modern foods are often laden with pesticides, artificial additives, and harmful chemicals. The ASTR Diet eliminates these toxins to protect your body.

R - Restorative: Every meal in this diet is designed to replenish nutrients, repair tissues, and support your body's healing mechanisms.

An Overview of What's Ahead

This book is your guide to understanding the ASTR Diet and implementing it in your life. Each section builds upon the last, leading you step-by-step toward a healthier future:

America's Health Crisis: 73% Sick from Malnutrition

We examine the concerning statistics surrounding America's diet and investigate how malnutrition is contributing to the rise of chronic diseases. Understanding the full scope of this issue is a critical step toward developing effective solutions.

The Poison in Our Food

From artificial additives to harmful chemicals, this section uncovers the hidden dangers lurking in everyday foods and how they impact your health.

Organic vs. GMO vs. Pesticides: What's the Difference?

You'll learn the key differences between these food categories and how to make the healthiest choices for yourself and your family.

What's Really on Your Food Label?

Decoding food labels can feel overwhelming, but this section provides a simple guide to understanding what you're really eating.

The Hidden Risks of Trendy Diets

Not all popular diets are created equal. We discuss the risks of following trends and why they often fail to deliver long-term health benefits.

Breaking Free from Food Addiction

Food addiction is real and often overlooked. This section helps you identify addictive patterns and provides strategies to regain control.

ASTR Diet: Eat to Heal

Here, you get a detailed breakdown of the ASTR Diet, including its principles, benefits, and practical tips for implementation.

Macronutrients & Micronutrients: How a Balanced Diet Helps Your Body

This part dives into the science of nutrition, explaining how proteins, carbs, fats, vitamins, and minerals work together to support your health.

The Benefits of Fasting

Fasting isn't just about weight loss. Discover how intermittent fasting can promote healing, balance hormones, and enhance longevity.

Hydration for Life, Tea for Health

Learn why proper hydration is crucial, discover the best water filters, and explore how herbal teas can provide additional health benefits.

Snack Smart

Healthy snacking can bridge the gap between meals and keep your energy stable. This section includes tips and ASTR-approved snack ideas.

3 Steps to Transform Your Health

Transforming your health doesn't have to be complicated. This section outlines three simple steps to kickstart your journey.

Addendum

The addendum serves as a quick reference and a practical toolkit, including:

- Key points for easy reference.
- Foods to avoid.
- Short shopping list.
- Full shopping list.
- A collection of ASTR-friendly recipes to help you get started.

Your Journey Starts Now

This book is more than a guide; it's an invitation to take charge of your health and unlock your body's potential to heal. The journey may seem daunting at first, but remember: every small step brings you closer to a healthier, more vibrant life. Let's get started.

America's Health Crisis: 73% Sick from Malnutrition

Overweight (malnutrition) Epidemic

Overweight and obesity are often misunderstood as a result of excessive nutrition; however, they are, in fact, forms of malnutrition. Malnutrition is defined as an imbalance in nutrient intake, encompassing both deficiencies and excesses. Being overweight often stems from consuming diets high in calories but low in essential nutrients, such as vitamins, minerals, and fiber. This imbalance leads to excessive fat accumulation while the body remains deprived of the nutrients necessary for optimal health. Over time, this nutritional deficiency combined with caloric excess contributes to chronic conditions such as diabetes, cardiovascular disease, and metabolic syndrome. Recognizing overweight as a form of malnutrition emphasizes the importance of focusing not just on calorie intake but on the quality and balance of nutrients in the diet to support overall health and well-being. Obesity and overweight are significant public health concerns in the United States, affecting a substantial portion of the population.

Definitions:
- Overweight: A body mass index (BMI) of 25.0 to 29.9.
- Obesity: A BMI of 30.0 or higher.
- Severe Obesity: A BMI of 40.0 or higher.

Prevalence Among Adults (Aged 20 and Over):
- Overweight, Including Obesity: Approximately 73.6% of adults were classified as overweight or obese during 2017–2018.
- Obesity: The prevalence of obesity increased from 30.5% in 1999–2000 to 41.9% in 2017–March 2020.
- Severe Obesity: During the same period, severe obesity prevalence rose from 4.7% to 9.2%.

Prevalence Among Youth (Aged 2–19 Years):
- Obesity: The prevalence of obesity among youth increased from 13.9% in 1999–2000 to 21.1% in 2021–2022.
- Severe Obesity: During the same period, severe obesity prevalence rose from 3.6% to 7.0%.

The Health Risks of Overweight and Obesity

Overweight and obesity significantly increase the risk of developing numerous serious health conditions, making them critical public health concerns. Excess body fat, particularly around the abdomen, is associated with chronic diseases such as type 2 diabetes, cardiovascular disease, hypertension, and certain types of cancer, including breast and colon cancer. Additionally, carrying excess weight places extra strain on joints, increasing the likelihood of osteoarthritis and mobility issues. Obesity also contributes to hormonal imbalances, respiratory conditions like sleep apnea, and mental health challenges, including depression and anxiety. The combination of these risks not only reduces quality of life but also shortens life expectancy.

Overweight and Obesity as Forms of Malnutrition

Malnutrition is typically associated with undernutrition, but it also encompasses overnutrition, including overweight and obesity. The World Health Organization (WHO) defines malnutrition as imbalances in a person's intake of energy and/or nutrients, which can manifest as both undernutrition (wasting, stunting, or deficiencies) and overnutrition (overweight, obesity, and diet-related noncommunicable diseases).

Why Overweight and Obesity Are Forms of Malnutrition

1. Imbalanced Diet:

Overweight and obesity are closely linked to an imbalanced diet that prioritizes calorie-dense, nutrient-poor foods. Consuming excessive amounts of refined carbohydrates, unhealthy fats, and added sugars while neglecting essential nutrients leads to weight gain and nutritional deficiencies. Diets high in processed and fast foods often lack adequate vitamins, minerals, fiber, and healthy fats, creating a paradox where individuals may be overfed in terms of calories but undernourished in essential nutrients.

This imbalance not only contributes to weight gain but also disrupts metabolic processes, exacerbating issues such as insulin resistance, chronic inflammation, and hormonal imbalances. Over time, these effects increase the risk of developing chronic conditions like diabetes, cardiovascular disease, and non-alcoholic fatty liver disease. Addressing overweight requires more than just reducing calorie intake; it demands a shift toward balanced, nutrient-dense meals that provide the body with the necessary fuel for optimal function. A well-rounded diet supports sustainable weight management, overall health, and the prevention of nutrition-related diseases.

2. Nutritional Deficiencies:

Despite the association of overweight and obesity with excess calorie intake, research has consistently shown that individuals in these categories often suffer from nutritional deficiencies. Studies reveal that diets high in processed and calorie-dense foods typically lack essential vitamins and minerals, leading to deficiencies even in those who are overweight or obese.

A. **Vitamin D Deficiency**: Studies indicate a strong correlation between obesity and vitamin D deficiency. Adipose tissue sequesters vitamin D, reducing its availability for metabolic processes. Low levels of vitamin D have been linked to inflammation, insulin resistance, and a higher risk of chronic diseases such as diabetes and cardiovascular issues.

B. **Iron Deficiency**: Obesity has been associated with impaired iron absorption, potentially due to chronic low-grade inflammation that alters iron metabolism. Iron deficiency can result in fatigue, decreased immune function, and reduced cognitive performance.

C. **Magnesium Deficiency**: Research shows that overweight individuals are more likely to have low magnesium levels, a mineral essential for muscle function, heart health, and blood sugar regulation. Deficiency in magnesium can exacerbate metabolic syndrome and insulin resistance.

D. **Zinc Deficiency**: Obesity has been linked to zinc deficiency, as higher levels of inflammation in obese individuals can interfere with zinc absorption. Zinc plays a critical role in immune function, wound healing, and hormonal regulation.

E. **B-Vitamins Deficiency**: Insufficient levels of B-vitamins, such as B12 and folate, are common among those who are overweight. These vitamins are essential for energy production, red blood cell formation, and DNA synthesis. Deficiencies can lead to fatigue, anemia, and neurological issues.

F. **Calcium Deficiency**: Studies also highlight a connection between obesity and low calcium intake. Calcium is essential for bone health and metabolic processes. A deficiency can lead to osteoporosis and contribute to weight gain by disrupting fat metabolism.

G. **Vitamin A:** Vitamin A is vital for maintaining good vision, a strong immune system, and healthy skin. Deficiency often occurs in overweight individuals due to low consumption of fruits and vegetables. Symptoms include night blindness, dry skin, and increased susceptibility to infections.

H. **Potassium**: Potassium is an essential mineral that helps regulate blood pressure, fluid balance, and muscle contractions. Deficiency, common among overweight individuals, is often caused by low intake of fruits and vegetables and high sodium consumption. Symptoms include muscle weakness, cramps, and elevated blood pressure.

I. **Omega-3 Fatty Acids:** Omega-3 fatty acids are crucial for reducing inflammation, supporting heart health, and enhancing brain function. Overweight individuals often lack these healthy fats due to diets high in processed foods. Symptoms of deficiency include increased inflammation, poor cognitive function, and a higher risk of cardiovascular issues.

These findings underline the paradox of being both overfed and undernourished, highlighting the importance of focusing not just on calorie reduction for weight management but also on improving the nutrient density of diets. A diet rich in whole, nutrient-dense foods is essential to addressing both overweight and nutritional deficiencies effectively.

3. Metabolic Disorders:

Overweight and obesity are strongly linked to the development of metabolic disorders, which are a cluster of conditions that significantly increase the risk of chronic diseases. Key metabolic disorders associated with excess weight include insulin resistance, type 2 diabetes, dyslipidemia, hypertension, and non-alcoholic fatty liver disease (NAFLD). These conditions are driven by the accumulation of excess body fat, particularly visceral fat, which disrupts hormonal regulation and promotes chronic low-grade inflammation.

Insulin resistance, a hallmark of metabolic syndrome, occurs when cells become less responsive to insulin, leading to elevated blood glucose levels and an increased risk of type 2 diabetes. Similarly, dyslipidemia, characterized by elevated triglycerides, low HDL cholesterol, and high LDL cholesterol, is more common in overweight individuals. Excess weight also places additional strain on the heart and blood vessels, contributing to hypertension, which is a key factor in heart disease and stroke. Additionally, overweight individuals are at a higher risk for NAFLD, where fat accumulates in the liver, potentially leading to liver inflammation, scarring, and long-term damage.These metabolic disorders not only reduce quality of life but also pose significant long-term health risks.

Dual Burden of Malnutrition:

The WHO describes the "double burden of malnutrition," where populations face both undernutrition and overnutrition simultaneously, often due to shifts toward highly processed diets. Overweight and obesity contribute to this dual burden.

Overweight and obesity are classified as forms of malnutrition because they reflect a chronic imbalance in energy and nutrient intake. Despite consuming excess calories, individuals with obesity may suffer from deficiencies in essential nutrients, leading to poor overall health. Addressing these imbalances requires dietary changes that prioritize nutrient-dense foods while reducing excess caloric intake.

The Addictive Nature of Refined Carbohydrates

Refined carbohydrates, such as white bread, sugary snacks, and pastries, are not only widely consumed but also highly addictive due to their profound impact on the body's physiological processes and brain chemistry. Understanding the mechanisms behind this addiction is critical for addressing the health challenges associated with refined carbs consumption. Below is a comprehensive explanation of how refined carbohydrates create a cycle of dependency.

1. Rapid Blood Sugar Spikes and Crashes

Mechanism: Refined carbohydrates lack fiber and other nutrients that slow digestion. As a result, they are broken down quickly, causing a rapid surge in blood sugar levels.

Physiological Response: In response to this spike, the pancreas releases a large amount of insulin to bring blood sugar back to normal. This sudden drop in blood sugar, known as a crash, often leaves individuals feeling fatigued, irritable, and craving more carbohydrates to restore energy.

Cycle: This pattern of spikes and crashes creates a vicious cycle, reinforcing the habit of turning to refined carbs for quick energy, which perpetuates dependency over time.

2. Activation of the Brain's Reward System

Dopamine Release: Refined carbohydrates stimulate the brain's reward system by triggering the release of dopamine, a neurotransmitter associated with pleasure and satisfaction. This response is similar to the effects of addictive substances, providing a temporary "high."

Reinforcement: Over time, the brain starts associating refined carbs with comfort and pleasure, reinforcing cravings and making it increasingly difficult to resist these foods. This leads to an addictive cycle where refined carbs become a go-to for emotional or energy needs.

3. Disruption of Hormonal Balance

Leptin Resistance: Refined carbs interfere with leptin, the hormone responsible for signaling fullness to the brain. Leptin is primarily produced by adipose tissue (fat cells). It is a hormone that plays a key role in regulating energy balance by signaling the brain to suppress appetite and increase energy expenditure. The hypothalamus in the brain responds to leptin levels to help control hunger and body weight. Chronic overconsumption of refined carbs can lead to leptin resistance, where the brain no longer effectively receives signals to stop eating. This results in overeating and a continuous desire for more food.

Ghrelin Activation: Ghrelin, known as the "hunger hormone," increases before meals and decreases after eating. Refined carbohydrates cause ghrelin levels to drop quickly after consumption; however, this effect is short-lived. The rapid digestion of refined carbs leads to a quick return of hunger, prompting the stomach to produce more ghrelin. This cycle increases the frequency of eating and intensifies cravings, particularly for sugary or starchy foods.

4. Development of Insulin Resistance

How It Happens: Frequent consumption of refined carbs causes repeated insulin surges. Over time, cells become less responsive to insulin, a condition known as insulin resistance. This forces the pancreas to produce even more insulin to regulate blood sugar levels.

Impact: Insulin resistance not only impairs the body's ability to manage blood sugar but also perpetuates cravings for quick-energy foods like refined carbs, as the body struggles to maintain energy balance.

5. Lack of Satiation

Fiber Deficiency: Unlike whole foods, refined carbohydrates are stripped of fiber, a critical component that promotes fullness and slows digestion. Without fiber, refined carbs are digested quickly, leading to hunger shortly after eating.

Outcome: This lack of satiation encourages frequent eating and overeating, further fueling the cycle of dependency on refined carbs.

6. Chronic Inflammation

Impact on the Brain: Refined carbs contribute to chronic inflammation in the body, including the brain. Inflammation can impair the brain's ability to regulate hunger and cravings, disrupting normal eating patterns.

Long-Term Effects: Chronic inflammation exacerbates hormonal imbalances, weakens self-control mechanisms, and makes cravings harder to resist, further deepening the cycle of addiction to refined carbs.

Why This Matters

Refined carbohydrates exploit the body's natural mechanisms for energy regulation and reward, creating a destructive feedback loop that reinforces cravings and dependency. Blood sugar fluctuations, hormonal imbalances, and dopamine-driven rewards work together to make refined carbs both physiologically and psychologically addictive. Over time, this dependency undermines healthy eating habits, promotes overeating, and contributes to weight gain, insulin resistance, and other metabolic disorders.

Breaking this cycle requires not only reducing refined carbohydrate intake but also adopting a diet rich in nutrient-dense, whole foods that provide sustained energy and balanced nutrition. This approach supports stable blood sugar levels, healthy hormonal function, and a more sustainable relationship with food, ultimately promoting long-term health and well-being.

In the following chapters, you will learn how to transition from relying on refined carbohydrates to enjoying a variety of delicious, nutrient-dense foods that support your overall health and well-being. You will discover practical strategies to make this shift easier, such as identifying healthier substitutes, planning balanced meals, and incorporating a diverse range of whole foods into your diet. Additionally, you will learn tips for overcoming cravings, reprogramming your taste buds, and finding satisfying, flavorful alternatives that keep you feeling full and energized.

The Poison in Our Food

Understanding food chemical approval processes is important for consumers and health-conscious individuals. Familiarity with the USA and Europe's approval systems fosters informed decision-making, enabling individuals to choose safer, healthier food options, align their choices with their values, and advocate for stronger health protections within food systems. Additionally, this knowledge empowers consumers to critically evaluate food labels and chemical approvals instead of assuming they are inherently safe.

Food Chemical Approval Processes: A Comparison of the USA and Europe

In the United States and Europe, the safety of chemicals used in food (such as additives, preservatives, or processing aids) is evaluated through specific regulatory frameworks. Here's an overview of the processes and chemical safety evaluations in each region:

Differences in Safety Approval Principles: Precautionary Principle vs. GRAS System

The safety approval processes for food chemicals differ significantly between the United States and Europe, primarily due to the underlying principles guiding their regulatory frameworks. Two prominent principles are the Precautionary Principle (common in Europe) and the GRAS System (used in the U.S.).

1. Precautionary Principle (Europe)

The Precautionary Principle is a regulatory approach that prioritizes public health and safety in situations where there is scientific uncertainty about potential risks. It is widely applied in the European Union (EU).

Key Features:

Risk Aversion: A food chemical or additive will not be approved unless its safety is conclusively demonstrated. If evidence is inconclusive or incomplete, approval is withheld or restricted.

Burden of Proof: The burden to prove safety lies entirely on the manufacturer or applicant.

Preventative Action: Regulatory decisions favor erring on the side of caution, even when there is no definitive evidence of harm.

Dynamic Review: Approved substances may face restrictions or bans if new evidence suggests potential risks. For example, titanium dioxide was banned in the EU in 2022 due to concerns over its genotoxicity and increased risk of cancer. Unfortunately, it is still used in the USA.

Advantages:

- Protects public health by prioritizing safety over uncertainty.
- Encourages rigorous scientific investigation before approval.
- Provides a robust framework to address emerging scientific evidence.

2. GRAS System (United States)

The Generally Recognized as Safe (GRAS) system is the foundational principle for food additive regulation in the United States, managed by the Food and Drug Administration (FDA). It focuses on existing evidence of safety and historical use.

Key Features:

Historical Use: A chemical is considered GRAS if it has a long history of safe use in food, such as salt or vinegar, or if scientific evidence broadly supports its safety.

Self-Determination: **Manufacturers can self-certify substances as GRAS without requiring FDA pre-approval**. They may voluntarily notify the FDA, but it is not mandatory.

Risk Assessment Focus: Unlike the Precautionary Principle, the GRAS system focuses on balancing benefits and risks, with **regulatory action only if harm is evident.**

Criticisms:

- Lacks transparency, as companies are not required to disclose self-determined GRAS findings to the FDA.
- May result in insufficient oversight for newer or lesser-studied substances.
- Reactive rather than preventive, as it often relies on post-market evidence to address safety concerns.

Key Differences Between USA and Europe:

Aspect	USA (FDA)	Europe (EFSA)
Philosophy	Benefit-risk analysis	Precautionary principle
Approval Speed	Generally faster	More rigorous and slower
Consumer Protection	Less restrictive for certain additives	More restrictive, favoring consumer health
Risk Assessment	Industry-conducted studies often accepted	Independent reviews are more common

Problems Related to Industrial Farming:

Industrial farming, also known as intensive or factory farming, focuses on maximizing production at a large scale. While it has increased food availability, it also poses significant environmental, social, and health challenges:

1. Environmental Problems

Soil Degradation: Intensive monocropping depletes nutrients, compacts the soil, and increases erosion, reducing long-term soil fertility.

Water Pollution: Runoff from synthetic fertilizers, pesticides, and animal waste contaminates rivers, lakes, and groundwater, causing dead zones in aquatic ecosystems.

Deforestation: Expanding farmland for industrial agriculture leads to deforestation, destroying habitats and contributing to biodiversity loss.

Overuse of Water Resources: High water demands for crops like almonds or livestock feed contribute to aquifer depletion and water scarcity.

2. Health Issues

Antibiotic Resistance: Overuse of antibiotics in livestock to promote growth and prevent disease creates resistant bacteria that can threaten human health.

Pesticide Exposure: Widespread use of chemical pesticides poses risks to farmworkers and consumers, potentially causing long-term health issues like cancer and hormonal disruptions.

Low Nutritional Quality: Mass-produced crops and livestock are often less nutrient-dense due to the emphasis on yield over quality.

Zoonotic Diseases: Crowded conditions in factory farms can lead to the emergence of diseases that jump from animals to humans.

3. Animal Welfare Concerns

Inhumane Conditions: Animals are often kept in overcrowded and unnatural environments, leading to stress, disease, and poor quality of life.

Ethical Issues: Industrial farming methods raise ethical questions about the treatment of animals as commodities rather than sentient beings.

4. Social and Economic Problems

Loss of Small Farms: Industrial farming drives small, traditional farms out of business, reducing rural livelihoods and communities.
Corporate Control: A few large corporations dominate the food industry, reducing competition and farmer independence.
Worker Exploitation: Farmworkers often face low wages, poor working conditions, and exposure to hazardous chemicals.

5. Biodiversity Loss

Monocropping Practices: Growing only one type of crop reduces biodiversity, making ecosystems more vulnerable to pests and diseases.
Impact on Pollinators: Pesticides and habitat destruction harm essential pollinators like bees, threatening food security.

Shifting to sustainable farming practices, such as organic farming, regenerative agriculture, crop rotation, and agroecology, can mitigate these problems while promoting environmental health and food security.

The Problem of Monocropping

Monocropping, the agricultural practice of growing a single crop over large areas of land, poses significant challenges to soil health and environmental sustainability:

1. Nutrient Depletion:
Monocropping continuously depletes soil nutrients by repeatedly growing the same crop, which extracts specific nutrients from the soil without replenishment. For example, corn heavily consumes nitrogen, while wheat depletes phosphorus. Over time, this practice leads to soil imbalance and reduced fertility, as the lack of nutrient diversity makes it increasingly difficult for plants to thrive without significant reliance on synthetic fertilizers.

2. Soil Erosion:
Monocropping often leaves soil exposed between planting cycles, increasing the risk of erosion. Without cover crops or diverse plant roots

to hold the soil together, wind and water strip away topsoil—the most nutrient-rich layer.

3. Dependency on Chemical Inputs:
To compensate for nutrient depletion, farmers often rely on synthetic fertilizers, which can disrupt natural soil ecosystems, leach into water sources, and contribute to pollution.

4. Environmental Unsustainability:
Monocropping significantly reduces biodiversity, weakening ecosystems and making them less resilient. The lack of diversity allows pests and diseases to spread rapidly, often necessitating the increased use of pesticides. Additionally, some monocrops, such as cotton and almonds, demand large amounts of water, leading to unsustainable irrigation practices and the depletion of local water resources.

Studies Show Our Food Is Losing Nutrients

The following studies highlight the devastating effects of monocropping on the nutritional value of our food, showing a marked decline when compared to the same foods grown decades ago. Monocropping, the agricultural practice of growing a single crop repeatedly on the same land, depletes the soil of essential nutrients over time. This depletion directly impacts the crops, as nutrient-deficient soil leads to produce with lower levels of vitamins, minerals, and antioxidants. These findings underscore the long-term consequences of prioritizing high-yield farming techniques over sustainable practices, which not only harm soil health but also compromise the nutritional quality of the food we consume. Addressing this issue requires a shift towards diversified farming and regenerative agricultural methods to restore soil vitality and improve the nutritional content of our food supply.

1. White and Broadley (2005):

This study examined historical data on mineral concentrations in fruits and vegetables in the U.K. from the 1930s to the 1980s. The analysis revealed significant declines in several minerals:

   Copper: Decreased by 76% in vegetables.
   Sodium: Decreased by 49% in vegetables.
   Potassium: Decreased by 16% in fruits.
   Iron: Decreased by 24% in fruits.
   Copper: Decreased by 27% in fruits.

These reductions suggest a trend of declining mineral content in produce over the examined period.

2. Thomas (2007): This review examined data from the UK's McCance and Widdowson's food composition tables between 1940 and 2002. The analysis indicated notable reductions in mineral content for various foods:

   Vegetables:
      Copper: Decreased by 76%.
      Calcium: Decreased by 46%.
      Iron: Decreased by 27%.
   Meat:
      Iron: Decreased by 54%.
      Copper: Decreased by 24%.
   Dairy Products:
      Magnesium: Decreased by 10%.
      Iron: Decreased by 62%.

Numerous studies have highlighted the decline in nutrient density of foods over the past several decades. This trend is attributed to factors such as modern agricultural practices, soil depletion, and the prioritization of crop yields over nutritional quality.

Nutrient Loss After Harvest

Post-harvest nutrient loss in fruits and vegetables is influenced by factors such as storage conditions, time elapsed since harvest, and produce type. Research indicates that significant nutrient degradation can occur from harvest to consumption.

Vitamin C Losses:

A general decline in nutrient content occurs after harvest, as demonstrated by a 2007 study reporting that vegetables can lose between 15% to 77% of their vitamin C within a week, depending on the type of produce. For instance, mature spinach may lose up to 80% of its vitamin C content within just three days post-harvest, highlighting the rapid deterioration of essential nutrients in fresh produce.

Factors Influencing Nutrient Loss:

After harvest, fruits and vegetables continue to respire, breaking down stored organic materials, which contributes to nutrient degradation over time. Exposure to heat, light, and improper handling further accelerates this loss, while proper storage conditions can help mitigate some of the nutrient depletion and preserve their nutritional value.

Mineral Content Decline:

Historical trends show declines in mineral concentrations in produce over time, largely attributed to soil depletion and modern agricultural practices. Additionally, proper storage conditions, such as maintaining optimal temperature and humidity, can help slow nutrient degradation. Understanding these factors is crucial for both consumers and the food industry to minimize nutrient loss from harvest to consumption.

Grain-Fed vs. Grass-Fed Livestock: A Comparison

Health Issues in Livestock Fed Grain Diets

1. Acidosis

Ruminants are a group of herbivorous mammals characterized by their specialized digestive system, which allows them to break down tough plant materials like cellulose. They have a multi-chambered stomach, typically consisting of four compartments: the rumen, reticulum, omasum, and abomasum. This unique structure enables them to ferment food with the help of microbes, regurgitate it as cud, and re-chew it to aid digestion. Examples of ruminants include cows, sheep, goats, deer, and giraffes. Their ability to convert fibrous plants into energy makes them an essential part of ecosystems and agriculture, as they can thrive on vegetation that other animals cannot digest effectively.

Cows are naturally designed to digest grass; however, high-starch grains such as corn and soy disrupt the pH balance of their rumen, leading to acid buildup. This imbalance can damage the rumen lining, causing ulcers, and increase the risk of bacteria entering the bloodstream, which may result in liver abscesses. Additionally, grain-based diets contribute to chronic stress and reduced immunity in cows. Studies, including one published in PubMed (2016), have shown that grain-based diets significantly increase the occurrence of acidosis compared to forage-based diets.

2. Bloat

Grain diets produce more gas during fermentation in the rumen, particularly when finely ground grains are used. This gas accumulation can lead to rumen distension, compressing other organs and causing significant pain or even death if left untreated. Chronic bloat not only impacts the well-being of the animal but also reduces growth rates and overall productivity. Research published in the *Journal of Animal Science* (2019) highlights that cattle fed grain diets are at a higher risk of developing frothy bloat compared to those on forage-based diets.

3. Liver Abscesses

Grain-based diets can lead to ruminal lesions, creating pathways for harmful bacteria such as *Fusobacterium necrophorum* to enter the bloodstream and infect the liver. This not only compromises liver function and overall health but also results in significant economic losses due to condemned livers at slaughter. A study published in the *Veterinary Science Journal* (2020) found liver abscess rates as high as 32% in grain-fed cattle, compared to less than 2% in grass-fed cattle.

4. Weakened Immune System

High-grain diets lack the diverse nutrients found in forage-based diets, which increases cattle's susceptibility to infections, leads to higher veterinary costs, and decreases overall productivity. A study published in *Frontiers in Veterinary Science* (2018) linked the nutritional deficiencies of grain-based diets to compromised immune responses in cattle. The findings highlight the importance of balanced nutrition for maintaining both health and performance.

5. Reproductive Issues

Imbalanced diets rich in grains can disrupt hormonal levels in livestock, leading to lower fertility rates and increased calving complications. A meta-analysis published in *Animal Reproduction Science* (2021) found that grain-fed livestock had significantly lower conception rates compared to grass-fed counterparts. This emphasizes the profound impact of diet on reproductive health.

The diet and growth management of livestock significantly influence their health, growth rates, and the time required to reach market readiness. Grain-fed livestock, often supplemented with growth hormones, exhibit different health outcomes and growth timelines compared to grass-fed animals.

6. Nutritional Differences:

Grass-fed beef typically has a lower total fat content and higher concentrations of certain vitamins, such as riboflavin and thiamine, compared to grain-fed beef. The choice between grain-fed and grass-fed livestock production involves trade-offs in animal health, growth rates, and meat nutritional content. While grain-fed cattle reach market weight faster, they may face health challenges related to their diet and hormone use. In contrast, grass-fed cattle have longer growth periods but align more closely with natural feeding behaviors and provide additional nutritional benefits.

Health Implications of Grain Feeding and Hormone Use:

The use of growth hormones in beef cattle production has raised significant environmental and health concerns. Studies have linked these hormones to the presence of potential endocrine disruptors in surface and groundwater, posing risks to aquatic ecosystems and potentially affecting human health through water contamination. Research published in *Environmental Health Perspectives* (2020) found measurable levels of hormone residues in agricultural runoff, which can disrupt hormonal balance in wildlife and humans. These findings underscore the broader implications of intensive cattle farming practices and the urgent need for sustainable and responsible agricultural methods.

Growth Rates and Time to Market:

Grain-Fed Livestock: These animals are typically finished on a high-energy, corn and soy-based diet in feedlots, allowing them to reach slaughter weight more quickly, usually between 15-18 months, at weights ranging from 1,200-1,500 pounds.

Grass-Fed Livestock: In contrast, grass-fed cattle continue grazing on pasture, reaching slaughter weight more slowly, typically between 20-28 months, at weights ranging from 1,000-1,300 pounds, depending on pasture quality and grazing management.

The Harmful Effects of Artificial Sweeteners

Artificial sweeteners are widely used as sugar substitutes in various food and beverage products. While they offer the advantage of reduced calorie intake, several studies have raised concerns about their potential health risks.

1. Cardiovascular Health Risks:

Research has raised concerns about artificial sweeteners and cardiovascular health. A study by the Cleveland Clinic found that elevated blood levels of erythritol, a commonly used artificial sweetener, were associated with a higher risk of major adverse cardiac events, such as heart attack and stroke. Similarly, research published in *The BMJ* indicated that higher consumption of artificial sweeteners in general was linked to an increased risk of cardiovascular diseases, including coronary heart disease and cerebrovascular disease.

2. Cancer Risk:

Aspartame and Acesulfame-K: The NutriNet-Santé cohort study suggested that consuming certain artificial sweeteners, particularly aspartame and acesulfame-K, is associated with an increased risk of cancer.

3. Metabolic Effects:

Some studies suggest that artificial sweeteners may negatively impact glucose metabolism, potentially contributing to insulin resistance and an increased risk of type 2 diabetes. For example, a study published in *Nature* (2014) found that certain artificial sweeteners altered gut microbiota in mice, leading to glucose intolerance. Additionally, human participants in the study exhibited similar metabolic changes when consuming these sweeteners. These findings highlight the potential metabolic risks associated with artificial sweetener consumption.

4. Neurological Concerns:

Recent research has explored the potential link between artificial sweeteners and mental health, particularly concerning the risk of depression. A study published in *JAMA Network Open* analyzed data from over 31,000 middle-aged women and found that higher consumption of ultra-processed foods, especially those containing artificial sweeteners, was associated with an increased risk of developing depression.

5. Gut Microbiota Alterations:

Research published in *Nature Medicine* examined the effects of artificial sweeteners on the gut microbiome and glucose tolerance. The study found that artificial sweeteners could induce glucose intolerance by altering the composition and function of the gut microbiota. These findings suggest a potential link between artificial sweetener consumption, changes in the microbiome, and negative impacts on metabolic health.

Another study, published in *iScience*, analyzed the impact of various non-aspartame artificial sweeteners on the small bowel microbiome. The research demonstrated that these sweeteners significantly altered the microbial community in the small intestine, indicating that artificial sweeteners can influence gut health.

Emerging research highlights potential health risks associated with the consumption of artificial sweeteners, particularly in relation to cardiovascular health, cancer risk, metabolic effects, diabetes, neurological concerns, and gut microbiota alterations..

The Hidden Harm in Processed Food

Food processing techniques can significantly impact the nutrient content of foods, often leading to the loss of essential vitamins and minerals.

The extent of nutrient degradation varies depending on the processing method, duration, temperature, and the specific nutrient involved.

Thermal Processing: Heat treatments such as pasteurization, blanching, and canning can degrade heat-sensitive vitamins, notably vitamin C and certain B vitamins. For instance, pasteurization of milk has been shown to reduce concentrations of vitamins B12 and E, while increasing vitamin A levels.

Blanching and Freezing: Food blanching is a cooking process where food, typically vegetables or fruits, is briefly boiled or steamed and then quickly cooled in ice water. Blanching vegetables before freezing can lead to nutrient losses; however, the subsequent freezing process helps preserve the remaining nutrient content. Studies indicate that while blanching may cause a 10% loss of vitamin C in peas, the freezing process itself does not significantly contribute to further losses.

Dehydration and Drying: Drying foods can result in the loss of heat-sensitive and water-soluble vitamins. The extent of nutrient degradation depends on factors such as temperature, duration, and the specific nutrient involved.

Food Enzymes:

Food enzymes are essential biological catalysts that facilitate the breakdown of nutrients in food, ensuring proper digestion and nutrient absorption. These enzymes are naturally present in raw foods and play a significant role in initiating the digestive process even before the body's own digestive enzymes take over. For instance, enzymes like amylase in fruits help break down carbohydrates into simpler sugars, protease aids in digesting proteins, and lipase supports the breakdown of fats into usable fatty acids. Consuming enzyme-rich foods, such as raw fruits, vegetables, and fermented products, can support the body's digestive system, particularly when natural enzyme production declines due to factors like aging, stress, or poor dietary habits. Food enzymes not only improve digestion but also enhance nutrient bioavailability, contributing to overall health and well-being.

Heat can decrease or deactivate enzymes in food. Enzymes are proteins that facilitate biochemical reactions, and they are highly sensitive to temperature. Here's how heat affects food enzymes:

1. Heat Denaturation of Enzymes

Denaturation: Enzymes lose their three-dimensional structure when exposed to high temperatures. This structural change prevents them from functioning properly.
Temperature Thresholds: Most enzymes are inactivated at temperatures above 118°F to 140°F (48°C to 60°C). The exact threshold depends on the specific enzyme.
Irreversible Inactivation: Prolonged exposure to high temperatures, such as during cooking, pasteurization, or canning, leads to permanent loss of enzyme activity.

2. Impact of Cooking on Enzymes

Blanching: Commonly used for vegetables before freezing, blanching inactivates enzymes to prevent spoilage and color changes during storage.
Cooking: Boiling, baking, frying, or steaming food significantly reduces enzymatic activity, which is why cooked foods have fewer active enzymes compared to raw foods. Heat decreases the viability of natural probiotics in food. Probiotics are live microorganisms, primarily beneficial bacteria and yeasts, that support gut health. They are highly sensitive to heat, and their survival is significantly impacted during food processing or cooking.

How Heat Affects Natural Food Probiotics

1. Heat Sensitivity of Probiotics: Probiotics are generally killed or inactivated at temperatures above 115°F to 130°F (46°C to 54°C).

Different probiotic strains have varying heat tolerances. For example: Lactobacillus and Bifidobacterium are heat-sensitive. Saccharomyces boulardii (a yeast-based probiotic) is relatively more heat-tolerant but still vulnerable to prolonged exposure to high temperatures.

2. Thermal Processing:

Pasteurization: This process, used for dairy and juices, heats products to 161°F (72°C) or higher, effectively killing most live probiotics.
Baking or Cooking: When probiotic-containing foods (like yogurt or fermented dough) are exposed to high heat, the probiotics are destroyed.
Sterilization and Canning: These involve even higher temperatures, eliminating virtually all probiotics.

3. Freezing vs. Heating:

Freezing preserves probiotics as long as the storage temperature remains stable and the product does not undergo repeated thawing and refreezing. Heating, in contrast, irreversibly kills probiotics.

Yogurt: Heating yogurt destroys live probiotic cultures, such as *Lactobacillus acidophilus*. This is why labels often specify "live and active cultures" to indicate that the yogurt has not been heat-treated.
Kefir and Kombucha: These probiotic-rich beverages lose their probiotic benefits when pasteurized or boiled.
Fermented Vegetables (e.g., Sauerkraut, Kimchi): Heat-treated versions, such as canned sauerkraut, lack the probiotic benefits found in raw, unpasteurized versions.

Heat significantly decreases the viability of probiotics in natural foods. To preserve their benefits, consume raw or minimally processed probiotic-rich foods and avoid subjecting them to high temperatures during preparation or storage.

Pasteurized Dairy Exposed

Pasteurization, the process of heating milk to destroy harmful bacteria, has become a standard practice for ensuring food safety. However, this process also alters the natural composition of milk, leading to the degradation of essential vitamins, minerals, enzymes, and probiotics. These changes can significantly reduce the nutritional value of dairy products and make them harder for the body to digest. The following are major issues with dairy pasteurization:

1. Enzymes

Milk naturally contains a range of enzymes that aid in digestion and nutrient absorption. Key enzymes such as lactase, lipase, and phosphatase are sensitive to heat and are largely destroyed during pasteurization. Lactase, in particular, helps break down lactose, the sugar in milk. Without this enzyme, individuals may struggle to digest lactose, leading to discomfort and lactose intolerance. Phosphatase, another important enzyme, assists in the absorption of calcium and phosphorus. Its deactivation during pasteurization reduces the overall digestibility of these essential nutrients.

Lactase is responsible for breaking down lactose, the sugar found in milk and dairy products, into simpler sugars (glucose and galactose) for digestion. Lactose intolerance are influenced by genetic, cultural, and dietary factors, resulting in significant variability across populations. While humans are generally born with the ability to digest lactose, the sugar in milk, lactase production typically declines after weaning in most individuals, leading to lactose intolerance. However, genetic mutations in some populations have enabled continued lactase production into adulthood, a trait known as lactase persistence.

Research on Lactose Intolerance

A. Swallow DM (2003):
This study in *Annual Review of Genetics* estimated that 65% of the

global population experiences a natural decline in lactase production after weaning.

B. Ingram CJ et al. (2009):
Published in *Human Genetics*, this research found that African and Asian populations see a 70–100% decline in lactase production after childhood.

C. Mattar R et al. (2012):
Research published in *Clinical and Experimental Gastroenterology* found that lactase levels typically decline by 75–90% in non-persistent populations between the ages of 2–5. It also noted that symptoms of lactose intolerance often manifest later, depending on dietary habits and tolerance thresholds.

D. Pediatrics Meta-Analysis (2006):
This meta-analysis confirmed that lactase activity decreases in 65–75% of the population globally, with regional variations. In East Asia, the decline reaches 90–100%

Pasteurization, the process of heating milk to destroy harmful bacteria, also destroys many of the beneficial enzymes naturally present in raw milk, including lactase. Lactase is the enzyme responsible for breaking down lactose, the sugar found in milk, into simpler forms that the body can easily digest. This poses a significant issue because studies indicate that **70–90% of the global population loses the ability to produce lactase after early childhood**, a condition known as lactase non-persistence or lactose intolerance.

Without the enzyme lactase in pasteurized milk, individuals who are lactase intolerance are unable to properly digest lactose, often resulting in symptoms such as bloating, gas, diarrhea, and discomfort. In contrast, raw milk retains its natural lactase content, potentially aiding in lactose digestion for those with reduced enzyme production. This enzymatic destruction during pasteurization highlights the challenge faced by the majority of the population who cannot produce lactase, making it crucial to explore raw milk (where safely sourced and regulated) for better digestive health.

2. Vitamins

Pasteurization impacts the concentration and bioavailability of heat-sensitive vitamins in milk. Vitamin C, a vital antioxidant that supports immune function and collagen production, is especially vulnerable to heat. Studies have shown significant losses of this nutrient during pasteurization. Additionally, certain B vitamins, such as B6 and B12, can degrade during this process. Vitamin B12, essential for energy production and neurological health, becomes less bioavailable, reducing its effectiveness. While fat-soluble vitamins like A, D, E, and K are more heat-stable, the overall nutrient profile of milk is diminished after pasteurization.

3. Minerals

Minerals in milk, such as calcium, phosphorus, and magnesium, are essential for bone health, muscle function, and various metabolic processes. Although pasteurization does not completely destroy these minerals, it can alter their bioavailability, making them harder for the body to absorb. Calcium, for instance, may bind to other compounds in milk during the heating process, reducing its solubility and effectiveness in promoting bone health. Phosphorus, which works synergistically with calcium, may also be affected, further impacting bone and dental strength.

4. Probiotics

Raw milk is a rich source of probiotics, live beneficial bacteria that support gut health, enhance digestion, and strengthen the immune system. Pasteurization destroys these probiotics, eliminating their potential health benefits. Probiotics such as *Lactobacillus* and *Bifidobacterium* are highly sensitive to heat and cannot survive the pasteurization process. The absence of these bacteria in pasteurized milk means that it lacks the gut-healing and immune-boosting properties that raw milk provides. This loss is significant, as probiotics play a vital role in maintaining a balanced microbiome and reducing inflammation in the body.

5. Protein Denaturation

In addition to the destruction of nutrients, pasteurization also denatures the proteins in milk. Protein denaturation refers to the process in which a protein's natural structure, specifically its three-dimensional shape, is altered. High heat alters the structure of proteins like casein and whey, potentially making them harder to digest and absorb. This structural change can contribute to digestive issues for some individuals, especially those sensitive to dairy products. Furthermore, the denaturation process reduces the natural enzymatic activity in milk, further compounding its reduced digestibility.

Based on the above information, it becomes challenging to justify the consumption of pasteurized dairy products due to their reduced nutritional value. While pasteurization ensures the safety of dairy, it comes with significant trade-offs, including the loss of vitamins, reduced bioavailability of minerals, destruction of enzymes, and elimination of probiotics. These changes compromise both the nutritional content and digestibility of milk. Based on the above information, it appears that pasteurized dairy products may be transformed into an indigestible white fluid. If the body is unable to digest them properly, this could result in internal inflammation and potentially lead to gastrointestinal issues. For individuals aiming to maximize the benefits of dairy, exploring raw alternatives may offer a more nutrient-dense option. However, it is essential to source these products from a reputable provider.

How Switching to Raw Dairy Transformed My Health

I have severe allergies to pasteurized dairy products, which previously caused a variety of health issues, including headaches, bloating, heartburn, elevated blood pressure, and a rapid heart rate. These symptoms significantly affected my daily life and overall well-being. However, since transitioning to raw dairy products, which I now consume regularly, I have experienced a remarkable transformation. All of my symptoms have completely resolved, allowing me to enjoy dairy without any adverse effects. Similarly, my son faced similar issues, including diarrhea after consuming pasteurized dairy. Since switching to raw dairy, he has experienced no such problems. The natural enzymes and unaltered nutrients in raw dairy have proven to be a healthier and more compatible option for both of us.

How to Choose a Safe and Ethical Raw Milk Farmer

When selecting a raw milk source, it's essential to prioritize hygiene and ethical farming practices to ensure safety and nutritional quality. Look for a farmer who maintains strict sanitation standards during the milking and bottling processes, as this minimizes the risk of contamination. The cows should be grass-fed, as pasture-raised animals produce milk that is richer in nutrients and free from harmful residues. Avoid farms that use pesticide-treated feeds or synthetic fertilizers, as these chemicals can indirectly affect the milk's quality. Visiting the farm is a great way to observe cleanliness, animal welfare, and adherence to natural farming practices. By choosing a farmer who values sustainability and hygiene, you can enjoy raw milk that is safe, wholesome, and environmentally responsible.

Harmful Food Packaging Chemicals

Harmful chemicals used in food packaging can migrate into food products, posing potential health risks. These chemicals may be intentionally added for functional purposes or be unintentional contaminants. Plastic packaging can potentially leach harmful chemicals into food, especially when exposed to heat, light, or prolonged storage. These chemicals, used during the manufacturing of plastic, may contaminate food and pose risks to health. Here's an overview of some harmful chemicals commonly associated with food packaging:

1. Bisphenol A (BPA)

Bisphenol A (BPA), a chemical commonly found in polycarbonate plastics and epoxy resins, is often used to line metal cans and food containers. As an endocrine disruptor, BPA mimics estrogen and can interfere with the body's hormonal systems. Studies have linked BPA exposure to infertility, developmental problems, and an increased risk of certain cancers. Many countries have banned BPA in baby bottles and sippy cups due to its associated health risks. However, it remains permitted in some food packaging and can linings in the United States, raising concerns about ongoing exposure and its potential impact on public health.

2. Phthalates

Phthalates are chemicals added to plastics, such as PVC, to enhance flexibility and durability. They are also found in adhesives, inks, and plastic wraps. As endocrine disruptors, phthalates are associated with reproductive issues, developmental delays, and metabolic disorders. Certain phthalates, like DEHP, are restricted in the U.S. and EU due to their health risks. However, other types of phthalates remain in widespread use, posing ongoing concerns for human health.

3. Per- and Polyfluoroalkyl Substances (PFAS)

PFAS, often referred to as "forever chemicals," are used in non-stick and grease-resistant coatings found in microwave popcorn bags, fast-food wrappers, and pizza boxes. These chemicals persist in the environment and bioaccumulate in the human body. Exposure to PFAS has been linked to cancer, thyroid disorders, and immune system suppression. Although certain PFAS are being phased out, many alternatives still carry significant health risks, making them a continuing environmental and public health issue.

4. Styrene

Styrene is a chemical found in polystyrene foam, commonly known as Styrofoam, which is widely used in takeout containers and disposable cups. It is classified as a potential carcinogen, with studies linking exposure to an increased risk of cancer and nervous system damage. The International Agency for Research on Cancer (IARC) has classified styrene as a "probable human carcinogen," sparking ongoing debates about its safety and future use in food-related applications. While some regions have restricted or banned the use of polystyrene in single-use food containers, it remains widely used in many areas, including the United States. This continued use raises significant concerns about its potential health risks and environmental impact.

5. Heavy Metals

Heavy metals, such as lead and cadmium, are present in printing inks, dyes, and pigments used on food packaging materials. These metals can leach into food, especially when packaging is damaged or improperly handled. Exposure to heavy metals is associated with neurological damage, developmental issues, and kidney dysfunction. Although regulations limit the levels of these metals in packaging, contamination risks persist, particularly in low-quality or recycled materials.

6. Mineral Oil Hydrocarbons (MOH)

Mineral oil hydrocarbons (MOHs) are commonly found in recycled cardboard and paperboard used in food packaging. These substances can migrate into food, especially dry and fatty products, leading to potential ingestion. MOH exposure has been linked to liver damage and inflammation. The European Union has implemented stricter regulations to limit MOHs in food packaging, but concerns remain regarding their presence in certain materials.

7. Formaldehyde

Formaldehyde is present in melamine-based resins and adhesives often used in packaging materials. The World Health Organization (WHO) recognizes formaldehyde as a carcinogen, with additional risks of respiratory problems and skin irritation upon exposure. While its use is limited in many countries, formaldehyde-containing materials are still found in some packaging in the U.S., highlighting the need for more comprehensive regulations.

8. Chlorinated Paraffins

Chlorinated paraffins are used as flame retardants and plasticizers in food packaging materials. These persistent organic pollutants are linked to cancer and liver toxicity, posing significant health risks. While some countries have restricted the use of chlorinated paraffins, they continue to be used in various packaging applications in others, raising concerns about their long-term impact on human health and the environment.

9. Teflon: polytetrafluoroethylene (PTFE)

Teflon, a non-stick coating made from polytetrafluoroethylene (PTFE), is commonly used in cookware due to its convenience. While Teflon is specifically used for cookware, not food packaging, it is included here due to its widespread usage. Potential health risks arise when Teflon cookware is overheated or damaged. Teflon can release toxic fumes, causing polymer fume fever, a condition with flu-like symptoms. Historically, the production of Teflon involved perfluorooctanoic acid (PFOA), which is considered potentially carcinogenic to humans. The International Agency for Research on Cancer (IARC), part of the World Health Organization (WHO), has classified PFOA as "possibly carcinogenic to humans." Damaged Teflon coatings can release small flakes into food, raising concerns with frequent exposure. For those seeking safer alternatives, stainless steel and cast iron are viable options.

While food packaging is essential for preserving and protecting food, harmful chemicals can pose significant risks to health. Stricter regulations and innovations in safer packaging materials are needed to address these concerns.

Ultra-Processed Foods - Fast Food Exposed

Fast food is a prime example of ultra-processed foods (UPFs), which are industrially formulated products made primarily from refined ingredients, additives, and preservatives. These foods are engineered for convenience, extended shelf life, and improved taste. They often contain ingredients such as hydrogenated oils, high-fructose corn syrup, artificial flavors, and emulsifiers. Fast food items, such as burgers, fries, and soda, typically undergo extensive processing, stripping them of natural nutrients and replacing them with synthetic additives to improve texture and flavor.

Regular consumption of ultra-processed fast foods has been associated with a range of health concerns, including obesity, heart disease, diabetes, and metabolic disorders. These effects are largely attributed to their high calorie density, low nutrient content, and excessive levels of salt, sugar, and unhealthy fats. As a result, the reliance on fast food contributes to poor dietary quality and raises significant public health concerns. UPFs pose significant health risks. Below is an overview of the issues associated with ultra-processed foods:

1. Nutrient Deficiency

Ultra-processed foods (UPFs) are typically low in essential nutrients such as fiber, vitamins, and minerals, making them nutritionally inadequate. White bread and sugary cereals undergo processing that strips them of significant nutrients. This process removes essential dietary fiber and micronutrients found in their whole-food counterparts. Instead, UPFs are often high in empty calories, providing energy without the nutrients needed for overall health. This imbalance between calorie content and nutrient density contributes to poor dietary quality and long-term health risks.

2. Excessive Sugar, Salt, and Fats

Ultra-processed foods (UPFs) are often packed with ingredients that can pose serious health risks. For instance, added sugars are a common component, significantly contributing to obesity, type 2 diabetes, and dental issues. Examples include sugary sodas, candies, and baked goods. High sodium levels are another concern, as excessive sodium intake increases the risk of high blood pressure, heart disease, and stroke. Examples include packaged soups, chips, and processed meats. Additionally, UPFs frequently contain unhealthy fats, such as trans fats and excessive saturated fats, which are known to contribute to cardiovascular diseases. Together, these ingredients make UPFs a significant driver of chronic health conditions.

3. Calorie-Dense and Overconsumption

Ultra-processed foods (UPFs) are engineered to be hyper-palatable, making them irresistibly appealing and leading to overeating. Examples include chips, cookies, and fast food. Additionally, these foods often lack fiber and protein, meaning they don't satisfy hunger effectively. This lack of satiety encourages excessive consumption, contributing to calorie overload and poor dietary habits.

4. Linked to Chronic Diseases

Ultra-processed foods (UPFs) are strongly associated with the development of chronic health conditions. They are a significant contributor to the obesity epidemic, as they are high in calories but low in essential nutrients, leading to weight gain and poor dietary quality. Regular consumption of UPFs also increases the risk of metabolic syndrome, which encompasses type 2 diabetes, heart disease, and liver disorders, due to their poor nutritional profile. Furthermore, a 2018 study published in *BMJ* found that diets high in UPFs are linked to an increased risk of certain cancers, including breast cancer.

5. Gut Health Disruption

Ultra-processed foods (UPFs) negatively impact gut health due to their lack of dietary fiber and the inclusion of harmful additives. Fiber, which is essential for maintaining a healthy gut microbiota and supporting digestion, is largely absent in ultra-processed foods (UPFs). This deficiency deprives the gut of the vital nutrients it needs to function optimally. Additionally, additives such as artificial sweeteners and emulsifiers can disrupt gut bacteria, leading to inflammation and digestive issues, further compromising overall gut health.

6. Additives and Artificial Ingredients

The additives commonly found in ultra-processed foods (UPFs) can have harmful effects on health. Preservatives, artificial flavors, and colors, such as tartrazine (Yellow 5) and monosodium glutamate (MSG), have been linked to allergic reactions, hyperactivity in children, and long-term health risks. Stabilizers and thickeners, like carrageenan, may irritate the gut or trigger inflammation, potentially worsening digestive and overall health issues.

7. Environmental Impact

The production and packaging of ultra-processed foods (UPFs) have significant environmental consequences. Their production relies on resource-intensive industrial farming practices, including monocropping and long supply chains, which contribute to deforestation, biodiversity loss, and greenhouse gas emissions. Additionally, UPFs are often packaged in single-use plastics and non-biodegradable materials, contributing substantially to pollution and waste, further harming the environment.

8. Psychological Impact

The consumption of ultra-processed foods (UPFs) can also negatively impact mental health and psychological well-being. Their addiction-like properties are designed to trigger dopamine release, reinforcing dependency and cravings, which can lead to overconsumption.

Additionally, diets high in ultra-processed foods (UPFs) are linked to increased rates of depression and anxiety. This is likely due to the nutritional deficiencies and blood sugar fluctuations caused by these foods. Beyond mental health, UPFs pose numerous risks, including promoting overeating, contributing to chronic diseases, disrupting gut health, and harming the environment. Understanding these impacts is essential for making healthier dietary choices and supporting long-term well-being.

Alcohol Consumption

Alcohol consumption is associated with a range of health issues, and recent studies have provided insights into the risks associated with varying levels of intake.

Health Risks Associated with Alcohol Consumption:

1. Cancer: Alcohol is a known carcinogen linked to cancers of the breast, liver, colon, rectum, mouth, and throat. The U.S. Surgeon General has highlighted that even moderate drinking can increase cancer risk.

2. Cardiovascular Diseases: While earlier studies suggested potential cardiovascular benefits from moderate alcohol consumption, recent research indicates that any level of alcohol intake may increase the risk of heart disease and stroke.

3. Liver Disease: Chronic alcohol use is a leading cause of liver diseases, including cirrhosis and liver cancer. The risk escalates with higher consumption levels.

4. Mental Health: Alcohol use is associated with mental health disorders such as depression and anxiety. It can also impair cognitive function and contribute to the development of alcohol use disorders.

5. Increased Mortality Risk: Studies have shown it may increase overall risks of death and chronic disease. Emerging evidence suggests that any level of alcohol consumption carries potential health risks, particularly concerning cancer and cardiovascular diseases.

Amount of Consumption That Causes Health Issues:

Recent guidelines and studies have shifted towards recommending minimal or no alcohol consumption due to associated health risks.

No Safe Level: The World Health Organization states that there is no safe level of alcohol consumption, emphasizing that even low levels can increase health risks. Even moderate alcohol consumption carries significant health risks. The Centers for Disease Control and Prevention (CDC) defines moderate drinking as up to one drink per day for women and up to two drinks per day for men. Research indicates that even modest alcohol intake can increase the risk of developing certain cancers, including breast, liver, and colorectal cancers. Additionally, it has been linked to an elevated risk of heart disease and high blood pressure. Alcohol is a known toxin that disrupts cellular processes and damages tissues over time, even at low doses.

Additionally, moderate drinking has been linked to an increased risk of cognitive decline and impaired mental health. While the social and relaxation benefits of alcohol are often highlighted, it is important to acknowledge that no level of alcohol consumption is entirely safe. Complete abstinence offers the lowest risk for adverse health outcomes.

Seeds Oil Exposed

In the American diet, several seed oils are commonly used for cooking due to their affordability, availability, and high smoke points. These include canola oil (from rapeseed), soybean oil, sunflower oil, cottonseed oil, and safflower oil. Additionally, sesame oil is frequently used in Asian-inspired dishes, while grapeseed oil is popular for dressings and sautéing. These seed oils are widely incorporated into processed foods, frying, and home cooking, making them a staple in many American kitchens.

The extraction and refining of seed oils involve several chemical processes designed to maximize yield and improve product quality. Here's an overview of the key chemicals used and their potential health implications:

Chemical Processes and Key Chemicals in Oil Refining

1. Solvent Extraction

One of the primary methods for extracting oil from seeds is solvent extraction. This process uses hexane, a petroleum-derived solvent, due to its high efficiency in dissolving lipids. During the process, hexane is mixed with crushed seeds to separate the oil. The solvent is then removed through evaporation or distillation. While this process is effective, concerns exist regarding residual hexane in the final product.

2. Degumming and Neutralization

The degumming process involves the use of phosphoric acid to remove phospholipids and other impurities from crude oil. This step enhances the oil's stability and reduces the risk of spoilage, making it more suitable for long-term storage and consumption. Neutralization ensures that free fatty acids are removed, further refining the oil's quality. The degumming and neutralization processes in seed oil refining can pose health risks by removing beneficial nutrients such as antioxidants and phospholipids. These processes may also promote the formation of harmful trans fats and introduce chemical residues and oxidized compounds. These processes can lead to oxidative stress, inflammation, and increased risks of chronic diseases like heart disease and atherosclerosis.

3. Bleaching

To improve the appearance and oxidative stability of oils, bleaching clays such as bentonite are used. These clays remove pigments, trace metals, and oxidation products from the crude oil. This process results in a clearer and more visually appealing final product. However, this step can also strip some beneficial compounds naturally present in the oil.

4. Deodorization

Deodorization involves steam distillation at high temperatures to remove volatile compounds responsible for undesirable odors and flavors. This process ensures the oil has a neutral smell and taste, making it suitable for culinary uses. However, the high temperatures used during deodorization may lead to the formation of harmful compounds, such as trans fatty acids.

Potential Health Implications

Hexane Residues

While the refining process aims to remove hexane, trace amounts may remain in the final product. Studies show that residual concentrations in edible oils are typically minimal and unlikely to pose significant health risks. However, prolonged exposure to hexane has been linked to neurological effects, underscoring the need for stringent industrial handling protocols.

Trans Fat Formation

High-temperature processes, especially during deodorization, can result in the formation of trans fatty acids. These harmful compounds are linked to an increased risk of cardiovascular diseases. Although the trans fat content in most refined seed oils is relatively low compared to partially hydrogenated oils, it remains a potential health concern. This risk is particularly significant when these oils are consumed in large quantities.

Oxidation Products

The refining process often reduces natural antioxidants in crude oils, making the final product more susceptible to oxidation. Oxidized lipids can contribute to inflammatory responses and other health issues. Proper storage and handling, such as keeping oils away from light and heat, are essential to minimize oxidation and maintain oil quality.

The chemical processes involved in oil refining rely heavily on solvents, acids, and high temperatures to produce clear, stable, and neutral-tasting oils. However, these processes introduce potential health concerns, including residual hexane, trans fat formation, and oxidation products. Although regulatory measures are in place to minimize these risks, it is essential to recognize that these chemicals and processes are not entirely safe for human consumption.

Avoiding seed oils in your diet is a crucial step toward improving overall health. Seed oils, such as soybean, canola, and sunflower oil, are often highly processed and contain high levels of omega-6 fatty acids, which can contribute to inflammation when consumed in excess. Additionally, the refining process of seed oils often involves the use of chemicals, high heat, and solvents, which can produce harmful byproducts like trans fats and oxidized lipids.

Instead, opt for healthier alternatives like **extra virgin olive oil**, **avocado oil**, and **coconut oil**. Extra virgin olive oil is rich in monounsaturated fats and antioxidants that support heart health and reduce inflammation. Avocado oil offers similar benefits, with a high smoke point that makes it ideal for cooking. Coconut oil is higher in saturated fat but contains medium-chain triglycerides (MCTs). These fats are quickly metabolized and can serve as a steady source of energy. Choosing minimally processed, nutrient-rich oils enhances the flavor of meals while promoting better long-term health. These oils reduce exposure to harmful compounds commonly found in seed oils.

Farmed Fish Exposed

Farmed fish play a vital role in global aquaculture and include species such as catfish, salmon, tilapia, carp, trout, barramundi, bass, and pangasius. Aquaculture also encompasses various shellfish like shrimp, clams, oysters, mussels, and scallops.

Chemical Contaminants and Health Risks:

Studies have identified several chemical contaminants in farmed fish that pose potential health risks:

Polychlorinated Biphenyls (PCBs): Farmed salmon, in particular, have been found to contain higher levels of PCBs compared to their wild counterparts. These contaminants originate from the fishmeal and fish oil used in aquaculture feeds. PCBs are associated with various health issues, including cancer and immune system suppression.

Antibiotics and Pesticides: To manage diseases and parasites in densely populated farming conditions, antibiotics and pesticides are frequently used. Residues of these substances can remain in the fish, potentially contributing to antibiotic resistance and allergic reactions in consumers.

Microplastics: Research indicates that farmed fish may contain microplastics, which can accumulate through contaminated feed and the farming environment. The health implications of microplastic consumption are still under investigation, but concerns include potential toxicological effects.

Nutritional Differences: Farmed fish often have different nutritional profiles compared to wild fish, including higher fat content and altered ratios of omega-3 to omega-6 fatty acids. These differences can influence the health benefits typically associated with fish consumption.

Hydrogenated Fats Exposed

Hydrogenated fats, also known as trans fats, are commonly found in a variety of processed and packaged foods. These fats are produced through hydrogenation, a process in which hydrogen is added to liquid vegetable oils. This makes the oils more solid and stable, enhancing shelf life and improving texture. While partially hydrogenated fats were widely used in the past, their use has been restricted or banned in many countries due to health risks. Unfortunately, it is still used in the United States.

Hydrogenated fats are commonly found in a variety of processed and packaged foods. These include baked goods such as cookies, cakes, pies, pastries, muffins, and shelf-stable frostings. They are also present in fried foods such as French fries, onion rings, and fried chicken, especially from fast-food outlets. Snack foods such as packaged chips, crackers, and popcorn often contain hydrogenated fats. These fats are also commonly found in margarine, solid vegetable shortening, and non-dairy creamers. Additionally, processed foods such as frozen pizzas, pie crusts, and ready-to-eat meals often contain hydrogenated fats. Packaged mixes, including pancake, waffle, and cake mixes, may also include these fats. Extensive research has linked the consumption of trans fats to various adverse health outcomes:

1. Cardiovascular Disease: High intake of industrially produced trans fats is associated with a 21% increase in the risk of coronary heart disease and a 28% increase in mortality from such diseases.

2. Inflammation and Endothelial Dysfunction: Trans fats contribute to systemic inflammation and disrupt endothelial function, both of which play critical roles in the development of atherosclerosis. These effects significantly increase the risk of cardiovascular events.

3. Diabetes: Some studies indicate a link between trans fat consumption and an increased risk of type 2 diabetes. This may be due to their role in promoting insulin resistance.

4. Mortality: A comprehensive review indicated that high trans fat intake correlates with a 34% increase in all-cause mortality.

The consumption of hydrogenated and trans fats poses substantial health risks, particularly concerning cardiovascular health. Reducing or eliminating these fats from the diet is advisable to mitigate associated health hazards.

Gluten & Inflammation

What is Gluten and Why Is It Problematic?

Gluten is a protein complex found in wheat, barley, rye, and triticale. It plays a vital role in giving baked goods their elasticity and chewy texture. However, its structure makes it difficult for the human digestive system to completely break it down. In individuals with celiac disease, a genetic autoimmune disorder, or non-celiac gluten sensitivity (NCGS), gluten triggers an immune response that leads to inflammation and damage to the intestinal lining. This response can lead to symptoms such as bloating, abdominal discomfort, and diarrhea. It may also cause systemic issues, including fatigue, skin rashes, and joint pain. Even for individuals without these conditions, gluten's ability to increase intestinal permeability ("leaky gut") can contribute to low-grade, chronic inflammation. This inflammation may potentially worsen existing health conditions.

Health Risks Associated with Gluten-Induced Inflammation

In celiac disease, the immune system produces autoantibodies that target and damage the intestinal villi. These small, finger-like projections are essential for nutrient absorption. This damage results in malabsorption, leading to deficiencies in essential nutrients such as iron, calcium, and vitamin D. Consequently, it can cause conditions like anemia and osteoporosis. Moreover, prolonged inflammation in celiac patients has been linked to an increased risk of developing certain cancers, such as intestinal lymphoma. For individuals with non-celiac gluten sensitivity (NCGS), symptoms may not involve intestinal damage but can still trigger systemic inflammation. This inflammation can lead to fatigue, headaches, and worsening symptoms of other inflammatory conditions, such as rheumatoid arthritis or irritable bowel syndrome (IBS).

Foods That Contain Gluten

Gluten is a common ingredient in many staple and processed foods, including:

- Breads: White, whole wheat, multigrain, and sourdough.
- Pasta: Spaghetti, penne, lasagna, and other traditional wheat-based noodles.
- Snacks and Desserts: Cookies, cakes, pies, pretzels, and crackers.
- Condiments and Sauces: Soy sauce, gravies, salad dressings, and malt vinegar.
- Beverages: Beer, malted drinks, and certain flavored alcoholic beverages. Hidden sources of gluten can be found in processed meats, certain soups, flavored chips, and even medications or supplements. For those avoiding gluten, careful label reading is essential to identify and eliminate these hidden sources.

Healthier, Gluten-Free Alternatives

Fortunately, many nutrient-rich and naturally gluten-free foods are excellent replacements for gluten-containing products. Grains such as quinoa, millet, brown rice, amaranth, and buckwheat are packed with essential nutrients and provide versatile cooking options. Gluten-free flours, like almond, coconut, and chickpea flour, offer high-protein alternatives for baking. Additionally, whole foods such as fruits, vegetables, legumes, nuts, seeds, and unprocessed meats form the foundation of a healthy, gluten-free diet.

The Benefits of Reducing Gluten

Switching to a gluten-free diet can significantly reduce inflammation in individuals with gluten sensitivities, allowing the body to heal and thrive. Many people report improved digestion, increased energy, and enhanced mental clarity after removing gluten from their diets. For individuals with celiac disease, adhering to a gluten-free diet is not optional but a necessity. This dietary change is crucial to prevent long-term complications such as intestinal damage, nutrient deficiencies, and an increased risk of certain cancers.Even for individuals without diagnosed sensitivities, reducing gluten intake and prioritizing whole, nutrient-dense foods can support overall health. This approach may help minimize exposure to inflammatory agents and promote better gut health.

Peanuts and Aflatoxins

Aflatoxins are toxic compounds produced by molds, primarily *Aspergillus flavus* and *Aspergillus parasiticus*, which thrive in warm, humid conditions. These molds commonly contaminate peanuts during growth, harvest, and storage, especially when drying and storage practices are inadequate. Aflatoxins, classified as Group 1 carcinogens by the International Agency for Research on Cancer (IARC), pose serious health risks. These include liver cancer, immune suppression, and impaired growth in children. Chronic exposure to aflatoxins, even at low levels, is especially concerning for individuals with preexisting conditions like hepatitis B or C. This exposure significantly increases their vulnerability to severe health complications.

Aflatoxins pose a significant health concern in peanuts, particularly in regions where food safety measures are less stringent. A study published in the *Journal of Food Protection* revealed that over 50% of peanut samples tested in developing countries exceeded the European Union's maximum allowable aflatoxin limits (Otsuki et al., 2001). Long-term exposure to aflatoxins has also been shown to impair nutrient absorption, contributing to stunted growth in children (Williams et al., 2004). These findings underscore the critical need for effective monitoring and control of aflatoxin contamination in peanuts.

Although roasting peanuts can reduce aflatoxin levels, the process does not guarantee complete elimination, especially in heavily contaminated samples. Excessive heat during roasting can degrade essential nutrients, such as vitamins and healthy fats. It can also lead to the formation of harmful compounds like acrylamides, which have been associated with cancer risk and neurotoxicity (Magan & Aldred, 2007). Eliminating aflatoxins entirely from peanut products is challenging, and processing methods can introduce additional risks. As a result, limiting or avoiding peanut products may be a prudent choice for those prioritizing health and safety. Until more effective solutions for aflatoxin removal are developed, consumers are encouraged to exercise caution and prioritize alternative food options.

Organic vs. GMO vs. Pesticides: What's the Difference?

Genetically Modified Organisms (GMOs)

Genetically Modified Organisms (GMOs) are living organisms, including plants, animals, or microorganisms, whose genetic material has been artificially altered using genetic engineering techniques. This process involves altering an organism's DNA to introduce, remove, or modify specific traits. These changes enable characteristics that would not naturally arise through traditional breeding or natural evolution. GMOs are prevalent in various food products available in the market. Here's an overview of common GMO foods and their prevalence compared to non-GMO counterparts:

Common GMO Foods in the Market:

1. **Corn:** Approximately 92% of corn planted in the United States is genetically modified.
2. **Soybeans:** GMO soybeans constitute about 94% of all soybeans planted in the U.S.
3. **Cotton:** Around 96% of cotton planted is genetically engineered.
4. **Canola:** In 2013, GMO canola made up 95% of canola planted.
5. **Sugar Beets:** GMO sugar beets accounted for 99.9% of all sugar beets harvested in 2013.
6. **Papaya:** A significant portion of papaya grown in Hawaii is genetically modified to resist the ringspot virus.
7. **Alfalfa:** Genetically engineered alfalfa is used primarily for livestock feed.
8. **Squash and Zucchini:** Certain varieties have been genetically modified to resist viruses.
9. **Apples:** Specific GMO apple varieties have been developed to resist browning.
10. **Potatoes:** Some potato varieties have been genetically engineered to resist bruising and minimize the formation of acrylamide. Acrylamide is a potential carcinogen that can develop when potatoes are cooked at high temperatures.

Prevalence of GMO vs. Non-GMO Foods:

Processed Foods: It's estimated that approximately 75% of processed foods on supermarket shelves contain genetically engineered ingredients.

Market Share: While staple crops like corn, soybeans, and cotton have high GMO adoption rates (over 90%), other GMO foods like papaya, squash, and apples represent a smaller share of their respective markets.

Consumer Products: Many GMO crops are utilized in processed ingredients, including high-fructose corn syrup derived from GMO corn and soybean oil from GMO soybeans. These ingredients are commonly found in a wide range of food products.

Understanding the prevalence of GMO foods can help consumers make informed choices based on their preferences and dietary considerations. Additionally, awareness of the health effects of organic foods, genetically modified organisms (GMOs), and pesticide-treated foods is crucial. Here's a comparative overview based on current research:

1. Organic Foods:

Definition: Produced without synthetic pesticides, fertilizers, genetically modified organisms, antibiotics, or growth hormones.

Pesticide exposure is generally lower in organic produce compared to conventionally grown produce, with a Stanford University study revealing a 30% lower risk of pesticide contamination in organic options. Regarding nutritional content, some research suggests that organic foods may contain higher levels of certain nutrients. For instance, a systematic review indicated that consuming organic food might help reduce the risk of allergic diseases and obesity. In terms of microbial contamination, studies have found no significant difference in the risk of bacterial contamination between organic and conventional produce.

2. Genetically Modified Organisms (GMOs):

Organic vs. GMO vs. Pesticides

Definition: Organisms whose genetic material has been altered using genetic engineering techniques to introduce desirable traits.

One key concern about GMOs is their connection to pesticides. Many GMO crops are designed to be resistant to herbicides, such as glyphosate, allowing farmers to use these chemicals more liberally to kill weeds without harming the crop. Additionally, some GMOs, like corn, are engineered to produce their own pesticide within the plant, targeting pests directly. While this reduces the need for external pesticide applications, it raises questions about the long-term impact of consuming crops that produce pesticides internally.

3. Pesticides:

Definition: Chemical substances used to prevent, destroy, or control pests in agriculture.

Acute exposure to high levels of pesticides can cause immediate health effects, including respiratory issues, skin irritation, and neurological symptoms. Chronic exposure, even at low levels over time, has been associated with significant health concerns. These include cardiovascular diseases, adverse effects on the male reproductive system, nervous system disorders, and an increased risk of non-Hodgkin's lymphoma. When it comes to dietary intake, washing produce may not completely eliminate pesticide residues, as some can penetrate deeply into fruits and vegetables. While peeling can help reduce contamination, it may also remove beneficial nutrients, presenting a trade-off in maintaining food safety and nutritional value.

Pesticide Exposure and Cancer Risk

Pesticides have been linked to a variety of cancers, with the risk depending on the type of pesticide, cancer type, and level of exposure. Below is a detailed examination of the relationship between pesticide exposure and specific cancer types, supported by key studies.

1. Non-Hodgkin Lymphoma and Glyphosate

The French Cohort Study (2018) followed nearly 69,000 participants and revealed a significant finding. Those who consumed the highest amounts of organic foods had a 25% lower risk of developing cancer compared to individuals who consumed the least. The study found a 73% reduction in the risk of non-Hodgkin lymphoma among participants with the highest organic food consumption. Additionally, there was a 21% reduction in the risk of postmenopausal breast cancer in the same group. Research suggests a potential link between organic food consumption and reduced cancer risk.

A meta-analysis published in *Mutation Research* (2019) found a **41% increased risk of non-Hodgkin lymphoma** in individuals with high exposure to glyphosate-based herbicides. Glyphosate, widely used in agriculture, has also been associated with a higher prevalence of other cancers, such as multiple myeloma. These findings highlight the dangers of prolonged glyphosate exposure, particularly for agricultural workers who handle these chemicals regularly.

2. Prostate Cancer

Pesticide exposure has been strongly linked to prostate cancer, particularly among agricultural workers. Research in the *International Journal of Cancer* reported that certain pesticides are associated with a **14–35% increased risk of prostate cancer**. Additionally, a study identified 22 different pesticides that increased the risk, with four of them also raising the likelihood of mortality from prostate cancer. This underscores the need for protective measures for individuals in farming environments to reduce exposure.

3. Lung Cancer

Exposure to chlorpyrifos and other organophosphate pesticides has been associated with a **20–30% higher risk of lung cancer**, depending on the level of exposure. These findings are particularly concerning given the widespread use of these pesticides in both agricultural and residential settings. Such exposure highlights the potential for significant long-term respiratory health impacts, especially for individuals regularly exposed to these chemicals.

4. Leukemia in Children

Children are particularly vulnerable to the effects of pesticide exposure. A meta-analysis published in *Pediatrics* revealed that children exposed to household pesticides have a **47% higher risk of developing leukemia**. This alarming statistic highlights the importance of reducing pesticide use in homes and gardens. Prioritizing pesticide-free practices is especially crucial in areas where children are present to protect their long-term health.

5. Thyroid Cancer

Endocrine-disrupting pesticides have been linked to thyroid dysfunction and cancer. Research has shown that exposure to such pesticides is associated with a **33% increased risk of thyroid cancer**. These chemicals interfere with hormonal balance, potentially leading to abnormal cell growth in the thyroid. Individuals working in agriculture or consuming foods with pesticide residues may face greater risks.

6. Breast Cancer

Persistent organic pollutants (POPs), commonly found in pesticides, have been linked to an **18–50% increased risk of breast cancer**, as reported in environmental health studies. POPs accumulate in fatty tissues and persist in the body, creating long-term health risks. These findings suggest the need for stricter regulations on pesticide use and greater awareness of their potential impact on breast cancer prevalence.

The studies above illustrate the significant health risks posed by pesticide exposure, with clear links to various cancers, including non-Hodgkin lymphoma, prostate cancer, lung cancer, leukemia, thyroid cancer, and breast cancer. These findings emphasize the need to minimize exposure through dietary choices, protective measures for agricultural workers, and stricter regulations on pesticide use. Reducing reliance on chemical pesticides is essential for protecting public health and mitigating the long-term risks associated with these harmful substances.

Why Organic Produce Is Cheaper When Considering Health Costs

At first glance, organic produce might seem more expensive than GMO or pesticide-laden foods. When considering the long-term health effects of consuming pesticide-treated foods, the potential medical costs cannot be overlooked. Factoring in these expenses, organic produce becomes the more economical choice. The hidden costs of cancer treatments, including chemotherapy, radiation, and surgeries, far outweigh the upfront savings from cheaper, conventionally grown foods.

Pesticides used in conventional farming have been linked to an increased risk of various cancers, such as non-Hodgkin lymphoma, leukemia, and certain reproductive cancers. Continuous exposure to these chemicals, whether through food, water, or air, contributes to the development of chronic health issues over time. The financial burden of treating cancer is immense, with chemotherapy sessions often costing thousands of dollars each. Additionally, radiation treatments and surgeries require extensive resources, further adding to the overall expense. These medical costs can cripple individuals and families, far exceeding any savings gained from consuming cheaper, pesticide-laden produce.

Moreover, the physical and emotional toll of cancer treatments cannot be ignored. As a two-time cancer survivor, I have personally experienced the devastating effects of these treatments. My second cancer was a direct consequence of the treatment used to combat my first cancer, as the aggressive therapy that successfully eradicated the initial cancer inadvertently caused the second. Chemotherapy and radiation are not only expensive but also physically debilitating. Managing their side effects, such as nausea, fatigue, and weakened immunity, often necessitates additional medications and therapies, further increasing the overall burden. The loss of productivity and income during treatment further compounds the financial strain, creating an overwhelming burden for patients and their families.

By opting for organic produce, grown without synthetic pesticides and harmful chemicals, individuals can significantly reduce their exposure to carcinogenic substances and other toxins. This proactive choice may help prevent the need for life-altering medical interventions in the future. In contrast, organic farming prioritizes natural methods that protect both the environment and human health. By consuming organic foods, individuals invest in their long-term well-being, reducing the risk of chronic illnesses linked to pesticide exposure. This choice not only promotes a healthier life but also spares the financial and emotional burdens of treating preventable diseases. When factoring in the expensive cost of cancer treatments and their impact on quality of life, organic produce becomes a more affordable option. It stands out as a proactive and responsible choice in the long run. My journey has taught me the importance of prevention, and I firmly believe that prioritizing clean, chemical-free food can make a profound difference in reducing the risk of chronic illnesses, including cancer.

What's Really on Your Food Label?

How to Read Product Labels: Key Recommendations and Red Flags

Understanding product labels is essential for making informed and healthier choices. Below are key areas to focus on and the red flags to identify:

1. Chemicals and Additives

Product labels often include chemicals and additives that may pose health risks.

Preservatives to Avoid:
- Sodium Nitrite/Nitrate: Commonly found in processed meats; linked to increased cancer risk.
- BHA/BHT: Synthetic antioxidants that may disrupt the endocrine system.
- Propyl Gallate: A synthetic additive suspected of being carcinogenic.
- Artificial Colors (Red 40, Yellow 5, Blue 1): These frequently used dyes have been associated with hyperactivity in children and potential allergic reactions. Additionally, some studies have linked them to an increased risk of cancer.
- Artificial Sweeteners:: Aspartame, Sucralose, Saccharin: Linked to metabolic disorders and potential health risks.

2. Pesticides

Pesticide residues are a common concern in non-organic products and can pose potential health risks. To minimize exposure, look for certifications such as USDA Organic, which indicate lower levels of pesticide residues. Additionally, using resources like the "Clean 15" and "Dirty Dozen" lists can help identify safer produce options. Be cautious of labels with vague terms such as "natural" or "eco-friendly," as these often lack proper certifications and may not guarantee safety from pesticides.

The **"Clean 15"** and **"Dirty Dozen"** lists are annual reports published by the Environmental Working Group (EWG) to help consumers make informed decisions about their produce based on pesticide residue levels.

The Dirty Dozen: This list highlights the 12 fruits and vegetables with the highest levels of pesticide residues. These are the produce items that consumers are most often advised to buy organic to reduce pesticide exposure. Examples often include strawberries, spinach, and apples.

The Clean 15: This list identifies 15 fruits and vegetables with the lowest pesticide residues, making them safer choices when buying non-organic. Common examples include avocados, sweet corn, and pineapples.

Packaged Food Preservatives

Preservatives in processed foods can pose long-term health risks, making it essential to carefully examine ingredient lists. Ingredients like sodium benzoate, which has been linked to hyperactivity when combined with artificial colors, should be avoided. Additionally, potassium bromate, a known carcinogen banned in several countries but still permitted in the USA, poses significant health concerns.

Artificial Flavors

Artificial and vague flavoring terms on labels, such as "Artificial Flavor" or "Natural Flavor," can often conceal a mix of synthetic chemicals. These additives may lack transparency regarding their composition, raising concerns about their safety. To make healthier choices, prioritize products that list whole, recognizable ingredients over those with ambiguous flavoring terms.

Processed Fats

Processed fats, such as hydrogenated and partially hydrogenated oils, often contain trans fats. These fats are known to significantly increase the risk of cardiovascular disease. To make better dietary decisions, look for products labeled "No Trans Fats" or those listing 0 grams of trans fat on their packaging.

Serving Sizes and Hidden Sugars

Pay close attention to serving sizes on labels, as they can be misleading and result in underestimating calorie and sugar intake. Hidden sugars are commonly found in processed foods, often listed under names such as high fructose corn syrup, dextrose, maltose, or cane juice. Being aware of these terms can help consumers make healthier choices. To reduce sugar consumption, choose products with minimal added sugars and simple ingredient lists. Prioritizing whole foods is an effective way to support a healthier diet.

Tips for Spotting Red Flags

When evaluating food products, there are several red flags to watch for. Long ingredient lists, especially those with more than 10 unrecognizable names, often indicate highly processed items. Misleading claims, such as "natural" or "made with whole grains," should be cross-checked with certifications for authenticity. Always check for allergen warnings, particularly if you have sensitivities to gluten, dairy, or soy. Lastly, be mindful of products with extremely long shelf lives, as these typically contain heavy preservatives. By staying vigilant about these factors, you can make healthier and more informed food choices.

Making healthier choices starts with understanding product labels. Focus on avoiding harmful chemicals, choosing certified organic items, and selecting products with clear, minimal ingredient lists. This approach minimizes exposure to additives, pesticides, and synthetic chemicals, supporting long-term health.

What Do Produce Codes Mean?

Produce number indicators, also known as PLU (Price Look-Up) codes, are numbers found on stickers attached to fresh fruits and vegetables. These codes provide information about how the produce was grown and are standardized by the International Federation for Produce Standards (IFPS).

What the Numbers Mean:

1. Four-Digit Code (Conventional Produce):

Format: The code consists of four digits (e.g., 4011 for bananas).
Meaning: The produce was grown using conventional farming methods, which may include synthetic pesticides and fertilizers.

2. Five-Digit Code Starting with "9" (Organic Produce):

Format: The code begins with the digit 9 (e.g., 94011 for organic bananas).
Meaning: The produce was grown organically, without the use of synthetic pesticides, fertilizers, or GMOs.

3. Five-Digit Code Starting with "8" (Genetically Modified Produce):

Format: The code begins with the digit 8 (e.g., 84011 for genetically modified bananas).
Meaning: The produce was genetically modified (GMO).
Note: These codes are rarely used because GMO produce is often labeled differently, depending on regional regulations.

Examples of PLU Codes:

- **4011:** Conventionally grown bananas.
- **94011:** Organically grown bananas.
- **84011:** Genetically modified bananas (rarely seen in stores).

Understanding PLU codes can help consumers make informed choices about the type of produce they buy, whether they prefer conventional, organic, or GMO options. Not all produce items have a PLU sticker, such as bulk items or prepackaged produce. PLU codes are primarily intended for retail use and are not legally required to indicate organic or GMO status. To confirm the production method, look for additional certifications like USDA Organic.

Reasons to Choose Local Trusted Farmers for Produce and Meat

Freshness and Quality
Local farmers harvest produce at peak ripeness and deliver it quickly to markets, ensuring fresher and more flavorful food. Similarly, meat from local farmers is often minimally processed and handled with greater care. This attention to detail helps preserve its quality and taste, offering a superior alternative to mass-produced options.

Healthier Options
Local farmers are more likely to employ sustainable and organic practices, reducing exposure to harmful pesticides, hormones, and antibiotics. Smaller-scale farming often produces nutrient-rich fruits, vegetables, and ethically raised meat, offering healthier options for you and your family.

Transparency and Trust
Buying directly from local farmers allows you to ask questions about farming methods, ensuring the food meets your values and standards. Many farmers welcome visits, giving you the opportunity to see firsthand how crops are grown and animals are raised, fostering trust in your food source.

Supports the Local Economy
Purchasing from local farmers keeps money within your community, supporting small businesses and creating local jobs. It also strengthens

regional food systems, reducing reliance on industrial agriculture and promoting economic resilience.

Environmental Benefits
Local produce and meat require less transportation, significantly reducing carbon emissions and the overall environmental footprint. Additionally, many local farmers use sustainable practices that maintain soil health and promote biodiversity, contributing to a healthier ecosystem.

Ethical Treatment of Animals
Local farmers often prioritize humane treatment of livestock, offering free-range or pasture-raised conditions. These smaller-scale operations avoid the overcrowded and stressful environments common in factory farming, ensuring better welfare for the animals.

Seasonal Eating
Local farmers provide fresh, in-season produce, encouraging natural eating habits aligned with the growing cycle. This reduces reliance on imported, out-of-season products and promotes a healthier, more sustainable diet.

Emergency Resilience
Supporting local farms bolsters the local food supply, ensuring food availability during disruptions in global supply chains. A strong network of local farmers helps communities remain resilient in times of crisis.

Choosing local, trusted farmers for produce and meat offers multiple benefits. It not only enhances personal health but also promotes ethical practices, strengthens the local economy, and supports environmental sustainability. Making this choice builds stronger communities and fosters sustainable food systems.

How to Choose Local Farmers for Your Produce and Meat

1. Research and Recommendations

Start by gathering information about local farmers to ensure you find reliable and high-quality sources. Talking to neighbors, friends, or local food enthusiasts can provide valuable recommendations. Farmers' markets are excellent places to meet producers, ask questions about their practices, and explore their offerings. Additionally, online directories like **LocalHarvest.org** can help you locate nearby farmers and learn more about their farming methods.

2. Visit the Farm

Visiting a farm is one of the best ways to understand the farming practices and quality standards of a local producer. Many farmers offer tours where you can observe their operations firsthand. During your visit, pay attention to the cleanliness of the farm and ensure animals are raised in humane conditions..

3. Ask About Farming Practices

Asking farmers about their methods is essential to ensure the food aligns with your values. For produce, inquire whether they use synthetic pesticides or herbicides and whether they follow organic or sustainable farming practices. For meat and dairy, ask if the animals are pasture-raised, grass-fed, or free-range, and confirm whether antibiotics or growth hormones are used. This level of transparency is crucial for making informed decisions.

4. Check Certifications

Certifications provide reassurance that the food you purchase meets specific standards. Organic certification ensures adherence to strict organic farming practices. Non-GMO Project Verified labels confirm that crops or animal feed are free from genetically modified organisms, although they may still contain pesticides and synthetic fertilizers. Additionally, certifications such as Certified Humane, Animal Welfare Approved, or USDA Grass-Fed indicate ethical and sustainable practices for meat and dairy products.

5. Build Relationships

Establishing a strong relationship with your local farmer can help build trust and confidence in their products. Farmers who are transparent and open to discussing their methods are often the most reliable. Regularly purchasing from farmers who consistently maintain high-quality standards reinforces this trust and helps establish a long-term relationship with a dependable food source.

6. Read Reviews and Testimonials

Online reviews and testimonials from other customers can offer valuable insights into the quality and reliability of a farmer's products. These firsthand experiences can help you make informed decisions before committing to a particular producer, ensuring their practices align with your expectations.

7. Evaluate Pricing

Pricing is an important factor to consider when choosing a local farmer. Fair prices often reflect sustainable and ethical practices. Be cautious of prices that seem unusually low, as they may indicate compromises in quality or farming methods. Paying a slightly higher price often ensures better food quality and supports responsible farming.

8. Start Small

When trying a new farmer, start by purchasing a small amount of produce or meat to test the quality and freshness. This approach allows you to evaluate their products before committing to larger purchases. Starting small ensures you are satisfied with your choice and helps build confidence in your new food source.

By following these steps, you can confidently select local farmers who provide fresh, high-quality, and ethically produced food that aligns with your health and sustainability goals. Choosing local farmers involves research, relationship-building, and understanding their practices. By focusing on transparency, sustainability, and quality, you can find trusted farmers who align with your health and ethical values.

Cornucopia Institute

The Cornucopia Institute uses an ethical scale to evaluate and rate organic food products. The scale ranges from 0 to 5, with 5 representing the highest standard of organic and ethical excellence. It serves as a valuable resource for narrowing down which brands to purchase and identifying companies that uphold good ethical practices. For more information, visit: **www.cornucopia.org/scorecards/**.

What is Regenerative Farming?

Regenerative farming is an agricultural approach focused on restoring and enhancing the health of ecosystems through sustainable and holistic practices. Unlike conventional farming, which can deplete soil nutrients and harm the environment, regenerative farming focuses on restoring and improving soil health. It also promotes biodiversity and enhances water systems, contributing to a more sustainable agricultural approach. This method integrates practices such as crop rotation, cover cropping, no-till farming, agroforestry, and holistic grazing management to create a self-sustaining agricultural system.

The core principle of regenerative farming is to work in harmony with nature, promoting ecological balance rather than exploiting resources. It achieves this by enriching soil organic matter, enhancing biodiversity, and reducing reliance on chemical inputs such as synthetic fertilizers and pesticides. This approach provides a long-term solution to many environmental and agricultural challenges while ensuring food security for future generations.

Benefits of Regenerative Farming

1. Improved Soil Health

Regenerative farming replenishes soil nutrients and enhances soil structure by increasing organic matter. Practices like cover cropping and composting prevent erosion and improve the soil's water-holding capacity. Healthy soils support microbial activity, which promotes plant growth and reduces the need for synthetic fertilizers.

2. Enhanced Biodiversity

Regenerative farming creates habitats for a wide range of species, from soil microbes to pollinators and wildlife. Crop rotation and intercropping prevent monoculture farming and promote ecological diversity, which helps stabilize ecosystems and enhances resilience against pests and diseases.

3. Water Conservation

Healthy, nutrient-rich soils retain water more effectively, reducing runoff and erosion. This not only conserves water but also improves water quality by minimizing contamination from agricultural chemicals. Regenerative practices like holistic grazing also help restore natural water cycles in agricultural landscapes.

4. Resilience to Climate Extremes

Farms that implement regenerative practices are better equipped to withstand climate-related challenges, including droughts and floods. Enhanced soil health improves the farm's capacity to absorb and retain water, increasing resilience to extreme weather conditions.

5. Reduced Reliance on Chemicals

Regenerative farming reduces or eliminates the use of synthetic fertilizers and pesticides by promoting natural soil fertility and pest management. This not only lowers costs for farmers but also minimizes chemical runoff that can harm nearby ecosystems and human health.

7. Increased Nutritional Value of Food

Food grown through regenerative practices often has higher nutrient density because it is cultivated in nutrient-rich soils. This contributes to healthier diets and improved public health outcomes.

Regenerative farming is more than a sustainable agricultural method; it is a transformative approach aimed at restoring ecosystem balance. It addresses critical environmental challenges while promoting long-term resilience and sustainability. By improving soil health and promoting biodiversity, regenerative farming ensures long-term productivity and resilience. It offers a path toward a more sustainable future, where farming practices align with the natural world rather than deplete its resources.

The Hidden Risks of Trendy Diets

Popular Diets That Can Backfire

The Hidden Risks of Trend-Based Eating Plans

Many popular diets claim they reduce inflammation, improve energy, and promote rapid weight loss. In reality, most trending plans succeed short term because they reduce calories, eliminate ultra-processed foods, or simplify decision-making. However, many of these diets are built on restriction rather than restoration, and restriction often carries consequences that do not appear immediately. Over time, extreme dieting patterns can contribute to nutrient depletion, hormonal stress, gut microbiome disruption, elevated LDL cholesterol, loss of lean muscle mass, impaired metabolic flexibility, and higher long-term cardiometabolic risk (Mann et al., 2007; Seidelmann et al., 2018).

This chapter reviews common diets people follow for "health" and explains why these plans can create long-term harm, especially when used without clinical supervision or followed as a lifestyle.

1. Ketogenic (Keto) Diet

Principle

The ketogenic diet is a very low-carbohydrate, high-fat eating pattern designed to produce ketosis, a metabolic state where ketones from fat become a primary energy source.

Evidence-based concerns

Elevated LDL cholesterol and atherogenic risk

Randomized controlled feeding research in healthy, normal-weight women has shown that ketogenic diets can significantly increase LDL cholesterol, raising concern for atherosclerotic risk in susceptible individuals (Budoff et al., 2024). A 2024 meta-analysis of randomized clinical trials reported that ketogenic diets may increase total cholesterol and LDL cholesterol, even when weight loss occurs, reinforcing that weight loss does not automatically equal cardiovascular protection (Wang et al., 2024).

Liver dysfunction and fatty liver patterns

Long-term ketogenic feeding in animal models has been linked with hyperlipidemia and liver dysfunction, including fatty liver-like changes, suggesting that sustained high-fat intake may impair metabolic regulation in some settings (Gallop et al., 2025). While animal studies do not automatically translate to humans, these findings raise legitimate concern about long-term liver stress when diets are heavily fat-dominant.

Metabolic instability and long-term risk patterns

Low-carbohydrate extremes are associated with worse long-term mortality trends in observational data, particularly when carbohydrate reduction is replaced with animal fat and animal protein (Seidelmann et al., 2018).

2. Atkins Diet

Principle

The Atkins diet is a phased low-carbohydrate plan that begins with severe carbohydrate restriction and gradually increases carbs over time.

Evidence-based concerns

Long-term mortality associations in low-carbohydrate patterns

A systematic review and meta-analysis of observational studies found low-carbohydrate diets were associated with a higher risk of all-cause mortality (Noto et al., 2013). Another large cohort study and meta-analysis found increased mortality risk at both high and very low carbohydrate intakes, with the lowest risk at moderate intake levels (Seidelmann et al., 2018). These findings suggest that long-term extremes may carry unintended consequences.

Increased saturated fat exposure and LDL elevation risk

Low-carb diets often increase reliance on animal foods and saturated fat, which can elevate LDL cholesterol in many individuals, increasing atherosclerotic burden over time (Budoff et al., 2024; Wang et al., 2024).

Digestive consequences from fiber reduction

Carbohydrate restriction commonly reduces intake of fiber-rich foods such as legumes, whole grains, and certain fruits. Dietary fiber supports gut microbial diversity and production of short-chain fatty acids that regulate inflammation and metabolic health (Fu et al., 2022). Low fiber intake can contribute to constipation, gut irritation, and poor microbiome resilience.

3. Carnivore Diet

Principle

The carnivore diet eliminates all plant foods and relies entirely on animal-based foods, often including large amounts of red meat and saturated fats.

Evidence-based concerns

Severe fiber removal and microbiome disruption

Eliminating fiber removes a key fuel source for beneficial gut bacteria. Fiber fermentation supports production of short-chain fatty acids that influence gut barrier function, immune regulation, and metabolic health (Fu et al., 2022). Chronic low-fiber eating patterns can impair microbial balance and worsen inflammation signaling.

Cancer risk concerns from processed meat exposure

The International Agency for Research on Cancer (IARC) classified processed meat as carcinogenic to humans (Group 1) and red meat as probably carcinogenic (Group 2A), based on evidence linking meat intake to colorectal cancer risk (Bouvard et al., 2015; IARC, 2018). This is clinically relevant because many carnivore diets encourage frequent high-volume meat intake.

Higher type 2 diabetes risk patterns with red and processed meat intake

Large prospective cohort evidence and meta-analytic findings show red meat consumption, especially processed red meat, is associated with increased type 2 diabetes risk (Pan et al., 2011). This directly contradicts the claim that removing carbohydrates automatically protects metabolic function.

4. Paleo Diet

Principle

Paleo emphasizes meats, fish, vegetables, fruits, nuts, and seeds while excluding grains, legumes, and most dairy.

Evidence-based concerns

Short-term improvements do not equal long-term safety

A systematic review and meta-analysis found Paleo-style diets can improve metabolic syndrome markers in the short term, but the evidence base is limited and does not prove long-term safety or sustainability (Manheimer et al., 2015).

Nutrient restriction and long-term imbalance risk

Paleo eliminates multiple food groups that supply resistant starch, magnesium, and specific fibers. Long-term Paleo adherence has been associated with lower resistant starch intake, altered gut microbiota composition, and increased serum TMAO concentrations (Genoni et al., 2020). These shifts may negatively influence metabolic and cardiovascular risk over time.

Calcium deficiency risk

Excluding dairy can reduce calcium intake substantially, increasing risk for bone loss if not replaced with highly strategic food planning.

5. Whole30 Diet

Principle

Whole30 is a 30-day elimination plan removing grains, legumes, dairy, added sugars, alcohol, and additives, followed by reintroduction.

Evidence-based concerns

Unnecessary elimination can create deficiencies

Removing grains, legumes, and dairy at the same time increases risk of inadequate fiber, calcium, magnesium, vitamin D, and B vitamins unless carefully planned.

Restriction increases rebound risk

Highly restrictive diets frequently lead to a cycle of rigidity followed by overeating and weight regain. A major review found that dieting typically fails to produce sustained weight loss and can promote weight cycling and psychological burden (Mann et al., 2007). This pattern is especially common when diet structure depends on strict rules rather than sustainable biology.

6. Vegan Diet

Principle

Vegan diets eliminate all animal products, including meat, dairy, eggs, and fish.

Evidence-based concerns

Vitamin B12 deficiency is common without correction

B12 deficiency is consistently documented in vegetarian and vegan populations, often regardless of age or location, when intake is not specifically managed (Pawlak et al., 2013; Pawlak et al., 2014). B12 deficiency can lead to anemia, fatigue, nerve dysfunction, cognitive symptoms, and long-term neurological harm.

Fracture risk and bone integrity concerns

A large prospective study from EPIC-Oxford found that vegans had higher risks of total fractures and site-specific fractures, including higher hip fracture risk compared with meat-eaters (Tong et al., 2020). A 2025 meta-analysis also reported higher hip fracture risk in vegetarian and vegan patterns after adjustment for confounders (Ballarin et al., 2025). These findings strongly suggest long-term bone vulnerability when diets are not nutritionally corrected.

Protein and omega-3 limitations

Even when calorie intake is adequate, vegan diets can be insufficient in complete protein distribution and long-chain omega-3s (EPA and DHA), creating risks for lean mass decline, hormone disruption, and neuroinflammatory stress over time.

7. DASH Diet

Principle

DASH (Dietary Approaches to Stop Hypertension) emphasizes fruits, vegetables, whole grains, lean protein, and low-fat dairy while limiting sodium and processed foods.

Evidence-based concerns

Not metabolically protective in every patient

DASH has strong blood pressure evidence, but outcomes vary and can become problematic when the diet is implemented through processed grain-heavy "healthy" foods rather than truly whole foods (Filippou et al., 2020). In insulin-resistant individuals, a high-grain interpretation of DASH can worsen blood sugar volatility and appetite dysregulation.

It can still become a refined-carb pattern

DASH is often misunderstood as "low fat plus grains." When fiber quality is low and refined carbohydrates increase, metabolic markers may worsen rather than improve.

8. Detox and Juice Cleanse Diets

Principle

Detox and juice cleanses typically involve liquid-only intake, extreme calorie restriction, or "cleanse protocols" claiming toxin removal and rapid weight loss.

Evidence-based concerns

Little clinical evidence supports toxin-clearing claims

A critical review found very little clinical evidence to support detox diets for toxin elimination or sustainable weight management, despite widespread popularity and industry marketing (Klein & Kiat, 2015).

Microbiome disruption can occur quickly

A controlled dietary intervention study found that juice-based diets affected oral and gut microbiome composition differently than whole-food plant diets, raising concern about inflammation-linked bacterial shifts when fiber is removed (Sardaro et al., 2025). Northwestern University also reported microbiome shifts after just three days of juicing, emphasizing the risk of fiber-free diets (Northwestern University, 2025).

Blood sugar instability and muscle loss risk

Juice cleanses are typically low in protein and fiber and high in rapidly absorbed sugars. This combination promotes hunger cycles, glucose swings, fatigue, and loss of lean mass, especially in active individuals or those with insulin resistance.

9. Raw Vegan and Fruitarian Diets

Principle

Raw vegan diets emphasize uncooked plant foods, and fruitarian diets rely heavily on fruit as the dominant food source.

Evidence-based concerns

High risk of micronutrient deficiency long-term

A clinical review concluded that raw vegan diets exceeding 90 percent raw foods cannot be recommended long term due to micronutrient deficiencies and related complications (Pahlavani et al., 2023). These deficiencies commonly include B12, iron, zinc, iodine, calcium, vitamin D, and insufficient protein.

Bone fragility risk increases when protein and minerals fall

Bone outcomes in strict plant-exclusive diets are concerning when calcium, vitamin D, B12, and protein intake are not corrected (Ballarin et al., 2025; Tong et al., 2020).

Dental erosion and metabolic stress with high fruit intake

High-frequency fruit exposure increases acids and sugars against enamel, increasing risk for dental erosion and sensitivity over time in susceptible individuals.

Conclusion: Trend Diets Create Illusions of Healing

Most trend diets feel effective at first because they simplify eating and remove processed foods. But extreme restriction frequently creates long-term harm through nutrient depletion, gut dysregulation, metabolic instability, and cardiovascular strain (Mann et al., 2007; Seidelmann et al., 2018). True healing requires nutrition that supports the body's systems over time rather than forcing rapid weight changes through elimination, fear, or extremes.

Breaking Free from Food Addiction

Food addiction is a complex condition driven by a combination of psychological, physiological, and environmental factors. It is characterized by compulsive overeating and intense cravings, often for hyper-palatable foods rich in sugar, fat, and refined carbohydrates. Causes of food addiction can range from hormonal imbalances and nutritional deficiencies to emotional triggers and genetic predispositions. These factors work together to disrupt hunger cues, reinforce cravings, and create a cycle of dependency that can be difficult to break. However, with the right strategies, it is possible to overcome food addiction. By identifying underlying causes, adopting mindful eating practices, and fostering a supportive environment, individuals can regain control over their eating habits. This approach helps cultivate a healthier and more balanced relationship with food.

Psychological Causes

Food addiction is not solely a physical or physiological issue; psychological factors play a significant role in its development and perpetuation. These factors influence how individuals relate to food, often leading to compulsive eating behaviors that mirror patterns seen in other forms of addiction. Below are the key psychological causes of food addiction:

1. Emotional Eating

Emotional distress, such as stress, anxiety, depression, or loneliness, often drives individuals to seek comfort in food. Highly palatable foods rich in sugar, fat, and salt trigger the brain's reward system, temporarily alleviating negative emotions and providing a sense of relief or pleasure. Over time, this coping mechanism becomes ingrained, leading to compulsive eating whenever emotional distress arises.

2. Childhood Experiences

Early life experiences, including trauma, neglect, or exposure to unhealthy eating patterns, can predispose individuals to food addiction.

For example, comfort food associations formed in childhood, like receiving sweets as rewards, can lead to a lasting habit of seeking food for emotional gratification. These patterns may persist into adulthood, influencing eating behaviors. Similarly, individuals who have experienced abuse or neglect may use food as a coping mechanism to self-soothe and regain a sense of control. This behavior is perceived as helping them manage the emotional impact of trauma and stress.

3. Stress and Cortisol Dysregulation

Chronic stress elevates cortisol levels, a hormone that increases appetite and cravings for calorie-dense comfort foods. Consuming these foods temporarily alleviates stress by activating the brain's reward system. This creates a reinforcing cycle of stress-induced eating behaviors.

4. Poor Impulse Control

Impairments in the prefrontal cortex, the part of the brain responsible for decision-making and impulse control, can contribute to food addiction. Individuals with reduced self-regulation may struggle to resist cravings for highly palatable foods. This is especially true when they are exposed to environmental triggers, such as advertisements or social cues.

5. Body Image Issues

Individuals with low self-esteem or a negative body image may develop an unhealthy relationship with food. They might use it as a source of comfort or a way to escape from emotional distress. This behavior often becomes cyclical, as overeating leads to guilt or shame, which further drives compulsive eating.

6. Social and Cultural Influences

Social pressures and cultural norms can significantly contribute to food addiction. Social eating often leads to overeating, driven by peer pressure or cultural celebrations. This can contribute to normalizing excessive food consumption in such settings. Additionally, constant exposure to media and advertisements promoting unhealthy, hyper-palatable foods reinforces cravings. This perpetuates addictive eating behaviors makes it more challenging to maintain a healthy relationship with food.

7. Lack of Coping Mechanisms

Individuals who lack healthy strategies to cope with stress, boredom, or negative emotions are more likely to develop food addiction. Food becomes a default coping mechanism, reinforcing the behavior and preventing the development of healthier alternatives.

Biological and Genetic Causes

Genetics:

Research has shown that food addiction has a heritable component. Studies of families and twins suggest that genetic factors play a role in traits such as impulsivity, craving intensity, and sensitivity to food rewards. These traits are closely associated with food addiction. Genes linked to obesity and metabolic disorders, including those that regulate leptin, ghrelin, and insulin sensitivity, may contribute to the development of food addiction. These genetic factors can disrupt hunger and satiety signals, leading to impaired regulation of food intake.

Role of Specific Genes

DRD2 Gene: Variations in the DRD2 gene, which encodes dopamine receptors, have been associated with a higher risk of food addiction. Reduced dopamine receptor availability makes individuals more reliant on external stimuli, such as palatable foods, to experience pleasure.

FTO Gene: The FTO gene, commonly linked to obesity, is also implicated in food addiction. It may influence appetite control and food preferences, increasing susceptibility to overeating.

MC4R Gene: Variants of the MC4R gene, which plays a key role in regulating energy balance and appetite, have been linked to a stronger preference for calorie-dense foods. This genetic predisposition may contribute to the development of addictive eating patterns.

Hormonal Causes

Food addiction is strongly associated with hormonal imbalances, particularly involving leptin and ghrelin. These two key hormones play a central role in regulating hunger and satiety. Dysregulation of these hormones disrupts the body's natural hunger cues, resulting in overeating and increased cravings. This imbalance can also amplify the tendency toward addictive eating behaviors.

1. Leptin: The Fullness Hormone

Leptin is a hormone produced by fat cells that signals the brain when the body has had enough to eat. Its primary function is to suppress appetite and regulate energy balance. However, in individuals with food addiction or obesity, leptin resistance often develops, where the brain becomes less responsive to leptin's signals. Despite having adequate fat stores, the brain perceives a state of starvation. This misperception drives the individual to keep eating, even when they are not genuinely hungry. This creates a cycle of overconsumption and reinforces addictive eating patterns.

Leptin Resistance and Food Addiction:

In food addiction, leptin resistance reduces the brain's ability to recognize feelings of fullness, leading to compulsive eating. Individuals are often drawn to highly palatable foods rich in sugar, fat, or refined carbohydrates. Consuming these foods further disrupts leptin signaling, making it even harder to regulate hunger and satiety. This creates a vicious cycle, perpetuating overeating and worsening leptin resistance over time.

2. Ghrelin: The Hunger Hormone

Ghrelin is a hormone released by the stomach when it is empty, signaling the brain to stimulate appetite. It plays a key role in triggering hunger and motivating food intake. In food addiction, ghrelin levels can become dysregulated, resulting in heightened hunger and intense cravings. This often drives a preference for calorie-dense, hyper-palatable foods.

Ghrelin Overactivation and Cravings:

Frequent consumption of refined and sugary foods can heighten ghrelin sensitivity, making individuals feel hungrier more often. This exaggerated hunger response drives compulsive eating, even when the body has adequate energy stores.

3. Hormonal Dysregulation and Cravings

The interplay between leptin and ghrelin is critical for maintaining a healthy balance between hunger and satiety. In food addiction, the dysregulation of these hormones leads to persistent cravings and reduced satisfaction from meals. This drives a strong compulsion to consume foods that overstimulate the brain's reward system. This creates a vicious cycle where hormonal imbalances amplify cravings, reinforcing the addictive behavior.

Impact on Food Addiction

When leptin and ghrelin are out of balance, individuals lose the ability to accurately interpret hunger and fullness signals. This hormonal imbalance makes it difficult to resist cravings and manage portion sizes. The challenge is especially pronounced when exposed to highly palatable, addictive foods. Over time, this imbalance contributes to weight gain, emotional eating, and a worsening of the addictive cycle.

Brain Reward System

The brain's reward system plays a pivotal role in food addiction, particularly through the overactivation of dopamine pathways in response to highly palatable foods. These foods, often high in sugar, fat, or refined carbohydrates, stimulate the release of dopamine. This neurotransmitter creates feelings of pleasure and satisfaction, reinforcing the desire to consume these foods. While this mechanism is crucial for survival, as it drives eating and energy intake, it becomes problematic when overstimulated by hyper-palatable, calorie-dense foods. This overactivation can lead to compulsive eating and disrupt natural hunger regulation.

How the Dopamine Pathways Are Overactivated?

Palatable foods, such as sugary snacks, fast foods, and processed treats, are engineered to be intensely rewarding. When consumed, these foods flood the brain's reward centers with dopamine, providing an immediate sense of gratification. This surge is far greater than the dopamine release triggered by natural, whole foods. Over time, this heightened stimulation leads to desensitization, where the brain requires increasingly larger quantities of these foods to achieve the same level of pleasure. This phenomenon mirrors the mechanism seen in substance addiction.

Reinforcement of Addictive Eating Patterns

With repeated exposure to palatable foods, the brain begins to associate these foods with comfort, stress relief, and pleasure. This reinforces cravings and the habit of turning to these foods in response to emotional or environmental triggers, such as boredom, stress, or social cues. Over time, the drive to consume these foods becomes less about hunger and more about seeking the dopamine "high" they provide. This creates a cycle of compulsive eating, even when the body does not need the energy.

Impact on Self-Control and Regulation

Overactivation of dopamine pathways weakens the brain's ability to regulate self-control. The prefrontal cortex, a key area of the brain responsible for decision-making and impulse control, is significantly affected. Consequently, individuals find it increasingly difficult to resist cravings or make healthier food choices, further reinforcing addictive behaviors.

Long-Term Consequences

Chronic overstimulation of the brain's reward system by palatable foods can result in serious health consequences. These include obesity, metabolic disorders, and mental health issues such as anxiety and depression. The cycle of addiction often fuels emotional eating, where food is relied upon as a coping mechanism rather than for nourishment. This behavior further exacerbates the problem, creating a continuous loop of unhealthy eating patterns.

Habitual Behavior Causes

Food addiction is strongly tied to habitual behavior, as the repeated consumption of hyper-palatable foods can reinforce automatic eating patterns. Over time, these habits become deeply ingrained and challenging to overcome. These habits are reinforced by both psychological and physiological mechanisms, ultimately driving compulsive food consumption.

Formation of Eating Habits

Habitual behavior begins when actions, such as consuming specific foods, are repeated in response to certain triggers. For example, eating sugary or processed snacks while watching TV, during stress, or to celebrate can establish strong associations between those activities and food. Over time, these associations become ingrained, leading to automatic food-seeking behaviors, often without conscious thought or hunger.

The Role of the Brain

The brain plays a central role in habit formation, particularly through the basal ganglia, a region responsible for habitual actions. When hyper-palatable foods are consumed repeatedly, the brain's reward system strengthens these habits by releasing dopamine. This neurotransmitter is associated with feelings of pleasure, reinforcing the desire to continue consuming such foods. The more often these foods are consumed in response to specific cues, the stronger the neural pathways become, making the behavior feel natural and automatic.

Cue-Response Behavior: Triggers such as stress, boredom, or environmental cues (e.g., passing by a fast-food restaurant) can activate cravings. These triggers often lead to habitual food-seeking behaviors, reinforcing unhealthy eating patterns. These cues bypass decision-making processes, making it harder to resist eating.

Diminished Cognitive Control: As eating becomes habitual, the prefrontal cortex, which governs decision-making and self-regulation, loses its influence over these behaviors. This reduced control further reinforces the cycle of addiction.

Psychological Reinforcement

Habitual behavior is not just physical but also psychological. Eating hyper-palatable foods often provides emotional comfort, acting as a coping mechanism for stress, anxiety, or sadness. Over time, this emotional reinforcement strengthens the association between these foods and feelings of relief and comfort. As a result, breaking the habit becomes increasingly difficult.

Food Addiction Awareness

Food addiction is a complex condition characterized by compulsive consumption of palatable foods, particularly those high in sugar, fat, and salt. Individuals may engage in addictive eating behaviors with varying levels of awareness and self-control.

1. Addictive Behaviors with Lack of Awareness:

Some individuals may not recognize their compulsive eating patterns or the negative impact on their health. This lack of awareness can perpetuate the cycle of addiction. Studies indicate that people with food addiction often deny or minimize the consequences of their behavior, making intervention challenging.

2. Addictive Behaviors with Awareness but Lack of Self-Control:

Conversely, some individuals are aware of their unhealthy eating habits but struggle to exert control. This conscious inability to regulate food intake can lead to feelings of guilt and helplessness. Research indicates that food addiction shares key similarities with substance use disorders, involving the same brain regions and neurotransmitters. This overlap may help explain why exercising self-control in food addiction is so challenging.

Tips to Address Food Addiction

Overcoming food addiction requires a holistic approach that tackles the psychological, physiological, and emotional factors contributing to compulsive eating. This multifaceted strategy is essential for achieving lasting change and restoring healthy eating habits. Here are effective tips to help regain control and develop a healthier relationship with food:

1. Identify Triggers

- Understand Emotional Triggers: Recognize situations or emotions (e.g., stress, boredom, loneliness) that lead to overeating or cravings for unhealthy foods.

- Avoid Environmental Cues: Limit exposure to tempting environments, such as keeping unhealthy snacks out of the house or avoiding fast-food restaurants.

2. Prioritize Balanced, Nutrient-Dense Meals

- Incorporate All Macronutrients: Create meals with a balance of protein, healthy fats, and complex carbohydrates. This combination helps promote satiety and maintain stable blood sugar levels throughout the day.
- Focus on Whole Foods: Choose unprocessed, nutrient-dense foods such as vegetables, fruits, proteins, whole grains, nuts, and seeds. These choices help nourish your body and reduce cravings for unhealthy options.

3. Practice Mindful Eating

- Slow Down: Take your time during meals, savoring each bite and allowing your brain to register fullness.
- Eliminate Distractions: Avoid eating while watching TV or scrolling on your phone to prevent overeating.
- Listen to Your Body: Eat when you're genuinely hungry and stop when you're satisfied, not overly full.

4. Address Nutritional Deficiencies

- Check for Deficiencies: Work with a clinical nutritionist to identify and correct deficiencies in essential nutrients like magnesium, zinc, vitamin D, or omega-3 fatty acids.
- Supplement if Necessary: Use supplements under professional guidance to address persistent deficiencies that may drive cravings.

5. Manage Stress and Emotions

- Adopt Stress-Relief Practices: Incorporate stress-management techniques such as meditation, yoga, deep breathing, or journaling to reduce emotional eating.
- Seek Emotional Support: Talk to a therapist or join support groups to address underlying emotional issues that contribute to food addiction.

6. Create a Structured Eating Routine

- Set Regular Meal Times: Eating at consistent times helps regulate hunger hormones and reduces impulsive snacking.

7. Reduce Exposure to Hyper-Palatable Foods

- Limit Sugary and Processed Foods: Avoid foods high in sugar, salt, and unhealthy fats that overstimulate the brain's reward system.
- Replace with Healthier Alternatives: Satisfy cravings with nutrient-dense options like fresh fruit, dark chocolate, or nuts.

8. Build a Support System

- Involve Loved Ones: Share your goals with family and friends to create accountability and a supportive environment.
- Professional Help: Work with a nutritionist, therapist, or addiction specialist to develop personalized strategies for overcoming food addiction.

9. Be Patient and Persistent

- Understand the Process: Breaking food addiction takes time and effort, so be kind to yourself during setbacks.

- Focus on Long-Term Health: Shift your mindset from short-term gratification to long-term benefits, such as improved energy, mood, and overall health.

Addressing food addiction is a journey that involves self-awareness, consistent effort, and a supportive environment. By identifying triggers, focusing on balanced nutrition, and practicing mindful eating, you can regain control over your eating habits and build a sustainable, healthier lifestyle.

In the "3 Steps to Transform Your Health" chapter, overcoming addiction is simplified into an easy and fast approach. However, success relies heavily on the essential quality of self-control. Addiction, whether to unhealthy foods, substances, or harmful habits, thrives on repetitive behaviors and emotional triggers. Breaking free requires a conscious decision to prioritize health and long-term well-being over short-term gratification. While the method is straightforward and actionable, lasting success depends on your commitment to self-discipline and consistency in implementing these changes.

ASTR Diet: Eat to Heal

ASTR

The ASTR diet is founded on four core principles: Anti-inflammatory, Sustainable, Toxin-free, and Restorative. These principles are designed to promote overall health, prevent disease, and support the body's natural healing processes. The diet focuses on consuming whole, nutrient-dense foods that reduce inflammation, which is often at the root of chronic illnesses. It emphasizes sustainability, encouraging choices that are not only good for your body but also for the environment. ASTR eliminates harmful toxins found in processed and chemically-laden foods, replacing them with clean, natural options. Finally, it prioritizes restorative nutrition, providing the body with the essential vitamins, minerals, and nutrients needed for repair and optimal function. By following the ASTR diet, individuals can achieve lasting health and well-being.

ASTR Diet: Decoding the Abbreviation That Defines Health

The ASTR diet is a thoughtfully crafted nutritional approach built around four core principles: **Anti-inflammatory**, **Sustainable**, **Toxin-free**, and **Restorative**. Each component reflects a commitment to promoting health, preventing disease, and supporting the body's natural healing processes.

A - Anti-inflammatory
S - Sustainable
T - Toxin-free
R - Restorative

A - Anti-inflammatory: The cornerstone of the ASTR diet is its focus on anti-inflammatory ingredients. Chronic inflammation is a root cause of many health issues, including heart disease, diabetes, and autoimmune disorders. By incorporating foods known to combat inflammation, such as leafy greens, healthy fats, and antioxidant-rich fruits, the ASTR diet helps reduce systemic inflammation, improve cellular function, and promote overall wellness.

S - Sustainable: Sustainability is central to the ASTR diet, emphasizing the importance of choosing ingredients that are not only good for the body but also environmentally responsible. The diet promotes the use of local, organic, and minimally processed foods to minimize the environmental footprint. It also supports ethical agricultural practices by encouraging sustainable and responsible food choices. By aligning personal health with ecological well-being, the ASTR diet fosters a harmonious relationship between people and the planet.

T - Toxin-free: The ASTR diet prioritizes foods that are free from harmful chemicals, additives, and microplastics. Exposure to toxins through diet can contribute to a range of health issues over time. These may include hormonal imbalances and the development of chronic illnesses. The diet emphasizes clean, whole foods that minimize exposure to these harmful substances, creating a foundation for better long-term health.

R - Restorative: The restorative nature of the ASTR diet lies in its ability to nourish the body and support its natural healing processes. The diet provides a balanced intake of macronutrients such as fats, proteins, and carbohydrates, along with essential micronutrients. This combination helps rebuild and strengthen the body at a cellular level. Part of the ASTR diet is intermittent fasting, which supports tissue repair and metabolic optimization. This approach also helps maintain sustained energy levels throughout the day.

Together, these principles make the ASTR diet a comprehensive and holistic approach to achieving optimal health. It addresses both immediate nutritional needs and long-term wellness while promoting sustainability.

Building Your ASTR Diet Plate

The ASTR diet is a comprehensive nutritional approach that emphasizes variety, moderation, and balance by incorporating anti-inflammatory, non-toxic, and sustainable ingredients. This dietary framework is designed to support the body's natural healing processes while promoting long-term health. The diet divides each plate into equal portions: one-third fat, one-third protein, and one-third carbohydrates. This approach ensures a balanced intake of essential macronutrients. Every ingredient is carefully chosen to maximize nourishment and minimize exposure to harmful substances. Intermittent fasting is also integrated into the ASTR diet to enhance metabolic function, improve digestion, and support cellular repair. This holistic approach emphasizes nourishing the body with clean, healing foods. It also promotes sustainable practices that support both individual well-being and environmental health.

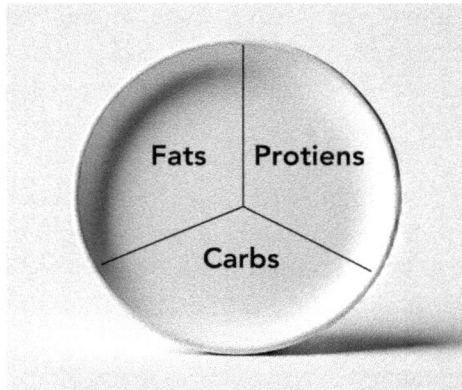

The Power of Balanced Meals in a Two-Meal Lifestyle

For the past seven years, I have followed a simple yet effective routine of eating two balanced meals a day, with no snacks in between. Throughout the day, I rely on water and tea to stay hydrated and energized. My first meal is in the morning before starting my day with patients, and my second is in the evening when I return home. What makes this routine sustainable is the effort I invest in crafting balanced meals. Each plate is thoughtfully prepared with one-third protein, one-third fat, and one-third carbohydrates to ensure the right proportions of macronutrients. This structure keeps me full, energized, and nourished, eliminating the need for snacks or additional meals. By focusing on balance and quality, I have been able to maintain this routine effortlessly, supporting my health and meeting the demands of a busy lifestyle.

On weekends, my eating routine adjusts slightly, as I typically enjoy my two meals within a 3-6 hour window during the middle of the day. This approach allows me to savor my meals within a shorter timeframe while maintaining a focus on balance and nourishment. Outside of this eating window, I stay hydrated by drinking water and tea. This helps me maintain my fasting routine during the remaining hours. This flexible yet mindful weekend routine complements my lifestyle and reinforces my commitment to intentional eating and overall well-being.

The Key to Sustaining the ASTR Diet: Enjoying What You Eat

For the past seven years, I have consistently enjoyed the first recipe in the recipe section. It perfectly aligns with the principles of the ASTR diet, offering a balanced, nutritious, and delicious option. Its great taste makes it easy to include in my daily routine, and I genuinely look forward to it. A key aspect of the ASTR diet is discovering foods and recipes you truly enjoy, as this fosters long-term adherence and satisfaction. When meals are both enjoyable and in harmony with the ASTR diet's guidelines, maintaining a healthy lifestyle feels effortless and sustainable.

The Importance of Timing Your Last Meal Before Bedtime

Eating and going to sleep immediately can harm digestion and overall health. I recommend leaving a 4-5 hour gap between your last meal and bedtime to promote better digestion and well-being. When you eat right before sleeping, your body is forced to focus on digestion rather than rest and recovery. This can potentially lead to issues such as acid reflux, indigestion, and disrupted sleep quality. Additionally, late-night eating can interfere with metabolic processes, increasing the risk of weight gain and elevated blood sugar levels over time. Allowing a 4-5 hour gap before bedtime gives your body enough time to properly digest your meal. This practice supports better sleep, improved metabolism, and overall well-being. This practice aligns with the body's natural circadian rhythm, allowing it to focus on repair and rejuvenation during sleep. By minimizing the energy-intensive process of digestion at night, overall health and recovery are enhanced.

Redefining Our Relationship with Food

Many people eat for the wrong psychological reasons, such as boredom or seeking comfort, rather than addressing genuine hunger. This mindset creates an unhealthy relationship with food, where eating becomes a source of distraction or entertainment instead of nourishment. The ASTR diet highlights the importance of eating only when you are truly hungry. This approach helps align your body's natural hunger signals with mindful and intentional food choices. One of its core goals is to encourage individuals to fully enjoy their meals when genuine hunger is present. This approach fosters a mindful and satisfying eating experience.By prioritizing nourishment and responding to genuine hunger rather than eating solely for enjoyment, the ASTR diet promotes healthier habits. This shift fosters a deeper appreciation for food and its role in supporting overall well-being.

Macronutrients & Micronutrients: How a Balanced Diet Helps Your Body

Good nutrition provides the body with essential nutrients necessary for energy, growth, repair, and overall health. Nutrients are classified into three main categories: macronutrients, micronutrients, and phytonutrients. Each plays a critical and complementary role in maintaining health.

1. Macronutrients: The Body's Essential Energy Sources

Macronutrients are nutrients required in large amounts that provide the body with the energy it needs to function and maintain overall health. They include carbohydrates, proteins, and fats, each playing distinct and vital roles in the body.

Carbohydrates: The Primary Energy Source

Carbohydrates are the body's main energy source, particularly for the brain and muscles. They can be classified into two types:

Simple Carbohydrates provide quick energy but often lack fiber and nutrients. Examples include table sugar, fruit juice, and candies.

Complex Carbohydrates offer sustained energy and are rich in fiber. Examples include whole grains like brown rice and oats, legumes such as lentils and chickpeas, and starchy vegetables like sweet potatoes.

For optimal health, focus on consuming complex carbohydrates and whole grains. Minimizing refined carbohydrates helps prevent blood sugar spikes and supports sustained energy throughout the day..

Proteins: Building Blocks of the Body

Proteins are essential for building and repairing tissues, producing enzymes and hormones, and supporting immune function. They are composed of amino acids, with essential amino acids being those that the body cannot produce and must be obtained through the diet.

Animal-Based Proteins include red meat, chicken, fish, eggs, and dairy.

Plant-Based Proteins include beans, lentils, quinoa, nuts, and seeds.

Quinoa is notable example of complete plant proteins, containing all essential amino acids. For a balanced diet, incorporate protein sources and mix plant-based and animal-based proteins.

Fats: Concentrated Energy and Essential Support

Fats serve as a concentrated energy source and are essential for maintaining cell membrane integrity. They also aid in the absorption of fat-soluble vitamins (A, D, E, K) and provide protection for vital organs.

Unsaturated Fats (Healthy Fats): Found in olive oil, avocados, nuts, and seeds, these fats promote heart health and reduce inflammation.

Omega-3 Fatty Acids: Omega-3 fatty acids, found in fatty fish like salmon and mackerel, as well as in walnuts and flaxseeds, are vital for brain health. They also play a key role in reducing inflammation throughout the body.

Saturated Fats: Found in red meat, butter, and full-fat dairy.

Trans Fats: Found in processed foods, these harmful fats should be avoided entirely.

To maintain a healthy fat intake, prioritize unsaturated fats and eliminate trans fats from your diet.

Macronutrients are the cornerstone of nutrition, each contributing to energy, structure, and overall health. By choosing nutrient-dense sources of carbohydrates, proteins, and fats, you can create a balanced diet that supports long-term well-being.

2. Micronutrients: Essential Vitamins and Minerals for Health

Micronutrients, including vitamins and minerals, are nutrients required in smaller quantities but are vital for numerous physiological functions. They play a critical role in energy production, immune function, bone health, and overall well-being. Below is a detailed explanation of key vitamins and minerals and their significance.

Vitamins

1. Vitamin A

Vitamin A is essential for vision, immune function, and skin health. It supports cellular growth and development, playing a critical role in maintaining healthy tissues. Dietary sources of this nutrient include animal products such as liver, eggs, and dairy. Plant-based options like carrots, sweet potatoes, and spinach provide it in the form of beta-carotene. Deficiency in vitamin A can lead to night blindness, dry skin, and weakened immunity.

2. Vitamin B Complex

The B vitamins play interconnected roles in energy metabolism, red blood cell production, and nervous system function. Vitamin B1 (thiamine) supports energy metabolism and can be found in whole grains, pork, and legumes. Vitamin B2 (riboflavin) aids in energy production and antioxidant function, with sources including milk, eggs, and leafy greens. Vitamin B3 (niacin) is essential for DNA repair and cholesterol regulation, found in poultry, and fish. Vitamin B6 (pyridoxine) supports brain function and hemoglobin production and is present in bananas, potatoes, and chicken. Vitamin B9 (folate) is crucial for DNA synthesis and pregnancy health, sourced from leafy greens and beans. Vitamin B12 (cobalamin) plays a key role in nerve health and red blood cell production and is found in animal products such as fish, meat, and dairy. Deficiencies in B vitamins can lead to symptoms such as fatigue, anemia, and neurological problems. In the case of folate deficiency, it may also result in birth defects.

3. Vitamin C

Vitamin C boosts the immune system, supports collagen synthesis, and acts as a powerful antioxidant. It is abundant in citrus fruits, strawberries, bell peppers, and broccoli. Deficiency in vitamin C can result in scurvy, characterized by gum bleeding, bruising, and weakened immunity.

4. Vitamin D

Vitamin D promotes calcium absorption for bone health and supports immune function. It is found in fatty fish like salmon and mackerel, and is synthesized through sunlight exposure. Deficiency in vitamin D can lead to rickets in children and osteoporosis in adults.

5. Vitamin E

Vitamin E protects cells from oxidative stress and supports skin and immune health. Its sources include nuts, seeds, and leafy greens. Deficiency in vitamin E can result in nerve damage and muscle weakness.

6. Vitamin K

Vitamin K is essential for blood clotting and bone health. It is found in leafy greens like kale and spinach, as well as broccoli and fermented foods. Deficiency in vitamin K can lead to prolonged bleeding and weakened bones.

Minerals

1. Calcium

Calcium is critical for bone and teeth health, muscle function, and nerve signaling. It is abundant in dairy products, and leafy greens. Deficiency in calcium can lead to osteoporosis and muscle spasms.

2. Iron

Iron is key for oxygen transport in the blood via hemoglobin. It is found in red meat, beans, lentils, and spinach. Iron deficiency can result in anemia, fatigue, and reduced immune function.

3. Magnesium

Magnesium supports muscle relaxation, energy production, and nerve function. It is found in nuts, seeds, whole grains, and dark chocolate. Deficiency in magnesium can lead to muscle cramps, fatigue, and irregular heart rhythms.

4. Potassium

Potassium regulates fluid balance, muscle contractions, and nerve signals. It is found in bananas, potatoes, spinach, and avocados. Deficiency in potassium can result in muscle weakness, cramps, and high blood pressure.

5. Zinc

Zinc boosts immune function, supports wound healing, and aids in cell division. It is found in meat, shellfish, beans, and nuts. Zinc deficiency can impair immunity and delay wound healing.

6. Selenium

Selenium acts as a powerful antioxidant and supports thyroid function. It is found in Brazil nuts, seafood, and eggs. Deficiency in selenium can weaken immunity and impair thyroid health.

7. Iodine

Iodine is crucial for thyroid hormone production and metabolism regulation. It is found in seafood. Deficiency in iodine can lead to goiter and hypothyroidism.

8. Phosphorus

Phosphorus is vital for bone health, energy storage, and cell membrane integrity. It is found in dairy, fish, poultry, and nuts. Deficiency in phosphorus can result in weak bones and fatigue.

9. Sodium

Sodium helps maintain fluid balance and supports nerve and muscle function. It is found in salt and seafood. Deficiency in sodium, or hyponatremia, can lead to confusion, fatigue, and muscle weakness.

Micronutrients are essential for maintaining optimal health and preventing diseases. Incorporating a variety of nutrient-rich foods into your diet provides your body with the essential vitamins and minerals it needs. This supports proper functioning and promotes long-term wellness.

Understanding Body Composition: The Building Blocks of Health

Body composition refers to the various components that make up the human body, including fat, protein, carbohydrates, water, and minerals. Each of these elements plays a critical role in maintaining physiological balance and supporting vital functions. By examining these components in detail, we gain a better understanding of how our bodies operate and how to optimize health and performance.

1. The Components of Body Composition

A. Fat

Fat is stored primarily in adipose tissue, located under the skin (subcutaneous fat) and around internal organs (visceral fat). It serves as the body's energy bank, providing a backup source of fuel when needed. Fat also plays an essential role in protecting organs, insulating the body, and producing hormones like leptin, which regulates hunger. Healthy fat levels vary by gender, typically ranging from 20–30% of body weight for women and 10–20% for men. While essential for survival, excessive fat storage, particularly visceral fat, is linked to increased health risks.

B. Protein

Protein forms the structural and functional backbone of the body, present in muscles, skin, hair, nails, and internal organs. Protein plays a crucial role in building and repairing tissues. It also supports the immune system by producing antibodies and facilitates chemical reactions through enzyme production. Protein makes up about 15–20% of total body weight, with lean muscle tissue being a significant reservoir. Foods rich in protein provide the amino acids necessary for tissue repair, enzyme production, and overall cellular function.

C. Carbohydrates

Carbohydrates are stored as glycogen in the muscles and liver and act as the body's primary quick-access energy source. Glycogen reserves make up only 1–2% of total body weight but are essential for energy. They play a critical role in fueling high-intensity activities such as running and weightlifting. Carbohydrates also provide the primary energy source for the brain. By breaking down carbohydrates into glucose, the body ensures a steady supply of fuel during periods of physical and mental exertion.

2. Tissue Composition

Different tissues in the body are composed of varying proportions of nutrients:

Muscle Tissue: Primarily made of protein and water, with smaller amounts of fat and glycogen. Muscles rely on carbohydrates and fats for energy, while protein is vital for growth and repair.

Fat Tissue: Composed of triglycerides, which act as the body's energy reserve. This tissue is utilized during fasting or prolonged exercise.

Bone Tissue: A combination of minerals, including calcium and phosphorus, and structural proteins like collagen. Bones require vitamins (such as vitamin D) and minerals for strength and maintenance.

Organs: Comprised of protein for structure, fat for energy storage, and carbohydrates for immediate fuel. These tissues rely on a balanced supply of nutrients to function efficiently.

3. Quick Summary of Energy Use

The body breaks down macronutrients differently to meet energy demands:

Carbohydrates: Provide quick energy for high-intensity activities and brain function.

Fat: Offers long-lasting energy for low-intensity and endurance activities.

Protein: Acts as a secondary energy source during crises and plays a vital role in tissue repair and immune function.

Body composition is more than just numbers; it reflects the intricate balance of nutrients needed for survival and optimal health. By understanding the roles of fat, protein, and carbohydrates, and how the body utilizes them, individuals can make informed choices. These decisions support physical performance, metabolic health, and overall well-being.

A balanced diet is essential for supplying the nutrients needed to maintain, repair, and support the body's tissues. Each type of tissue, including muscle, fat, bone, organs, and connective tissue, has specific nutritional requirements to function at its best. Meeting these unique needs helps promote overall health, optimize metabolic processes, and ensure the body performs efficiently.

1. Muscle Tissue

Muscle tissue is responsible for movement, posture, and generating heat. Its maintenance and repair depend heavily on the right balance of nutrients. **Protein** is essential for repairing and building muscle fibers, with sources including meats, eggs, quinoa, and lentils. **Carbohydrates** replenish glycogen stores, providing energy during physical activity, and are found in whole grains, fruits, and starchy vegetables. **Healthy fats** support prolonged activity and serve as an energy reserve, with examples including nuts, seeds, and avocados. Without adequate protein, muscles cannot repair after exercise or injury. Similarly, insufficient carbohydrate intake can lead to fatigue, while inadequate fat consumption limits long-term energy availability. This highlights the importance of balanced nutrition for supporting muscle health and overall energy levels.

2. Fat Tissue

Fat tissue plays a critical role in storing energy, insulating the body, and protecting vital organs. The consumption of **healthy fats**, such as those found in olive oil, fatty fish, and flaxseeds, provides essential fatty acids and energy. Additionally, **antioxidants** from foods like berries, spinach, and green tea help reduce inflammation within fat tissue. Excessive consumption of unhealthy fats, such as trans fats, can lead to chronic diseases and inflammation. On the other hand, inadequate fat intake can compromise hormone production and energy storage. This underscores the importance of moderation and choosing high-quality sources of dietary fat.

3. Bone Tissue

Bone tissue provides structure, protects organs, and serves as a reservoir for minerals like calcium and phosphorus. **Calcium**, found in dairy products and kale, is crucial for building and maintaining bone density. **Vitamin D**, obtained from fatty fish, and sunlight exposure, enhances calcium absorption. Additionally, **protein** supports the collagen framework within bones, with sources including eggs, meats, and beans. A diet lacking sufficient calcium and vitamin D can weaken bones, raising the risk of fractures and osteoporosis. Additionally, adequate protein intake is crucial for maintaining bone strength and integrity.

4. Organ Tissue

Organs are responsible for vital functions such as pumping blood (heart), filtering waste (kidneys), and digesting food (stomach). Nutritional support is key for optimal organ function. **Micronutrients** like **iron**, found in red meat, spinach, and lentils, are essential for oxygen transport. **Potassium**, sourced from bananas, sweet potatoes, and oranges, plays a key role in maintaining fluid balance. **Carbohydrates** provide quick energy for organ activity and are sourced from whole grains, fruits, and vegetables. **Healthy fats**, found in nuts, seeds, and avocados, maintain cellular membranes. Deficiencies in these nutrients can impair organ function, with iron deficiency leading to anemia and insufficient potassium causing muscle weakness and electrolyte imbalances. These imbalances can negatively impact overall health and well-being.

5. Skin and Connective Tissue

The skin serves as a protective barrier, while connective tissues like tendons and ligaments provide structural support and elasticity. **Vitamin C**, which promotes collagen production, is essential for maintaining the health of these tissues. Vitamin C, found in citrus fruits, bell peppers, and strawberries, is essential for maintaining skin integrity. It also supports the repair and resilience of connective tissues. Without adequate vitamin C, the body may struggle with wound healing and maintaining the structural integrity of skin and connective tissues.

Each type of body tissue has specific nutritional requirements, and a balanced diet ensures these needs are met. From protein and carbohydrates for muscle repair and energy to calcium and vitamin D for bone health, the proper intake of essential nutrients is crucial for overall well-being. These nutrients work together to support various bodily functions and maintain optimal health. Neglecting these requirements can lead to compromised tissue function, chronic diseases, and reduced quality of life. Prioritizing nutrient-rich foods tailored to the body's needs supports tissue health, promotes recovery, and sustains optimal physical and metabolic performance.

Phytonutrients: Nature's Powerful Compounds

Phytonutrients, also known as phytochemicals, are natural compounds found in plants that provide numerous health benefits beyond basic nutrition. While they are not considered essential nutrients like vitamins or minerals, they play a significant role in promoting health and protecting against chronic diseases. Phytonutrients are responsible for the vibrant colors, flavors, and aromas of fruits, vegetables, herbs, and other plant-based foods.

Categories and Examples of Phytonutrients

1. Flavonoids

Flavonoids are a large group of phytonutrients found in a variety of fruits, vegetables, and beverages like tea. Examples include quercetin in apples, anthocyanins in blueberries, and catechins in green tea. Flavonoids are known for their powerful antioxidant properties, which help reduce oxidative stress, support heart health, and lower the risk of certain cancers.

2. Carotenoids

Carotenoids are pigments that give red, orange, and yellow hues to foods like carrots, sweet potatoes, and tomatoes. Examples include beta-carotene, lutein, and lycopene. These compounds support eye health, boost immune function, and reduce the risk of chronic diseases such as cardiovascular disease. Beta-carotene, for instance, is a precursor to vitamin A, which is essential for vision and skin health.

3. Polyphenols

Polyphenols are abundant in foods such as berries, nuts, and dark chocolate. Examples include resveratrol in red grapes and ellagic acid in pomegranates. Polyphenols have anti-inflammatory and antioxidant properties that protect against diabetes, heart disease, and neurodegenerative disorders. They also promote gut health by supporting a healthy microbiome.

4. Glucosinolates

Glucosinolates are sulfur-containing compounds found in cruciferous vegetables like broccoli, kale, and Brussels sprouts. When consumed, these foods are broken down into bioactive compounds like sulforaphane. This compound has been linked to cancer prevention and supporting the body's detoxification processes..

5. Saponins

Saponins are found in legumes like beans, lentils, and chickpeas. They exhibit cholesterol-lowering effects, support immune function, and have potential anti-cancer properties by interfering with tumor growth.

Health Benefits of Phytonutrients

Phytonutrients contribute to health in several ways, including:

1. Antioxidant Protection

Phytonutrients neutralize free radicals, reducing oxidative stress that can damage cells and contribute to chronic diseases like cancer and cardiovascular disease.

2. Anti-Inflammatory Effects

Many phytonutrients, such as flavonoids and polyphenols, reduce inflammation in the body. Chronic inflammation is a risk factor for conditions such as arthritis, diabetes, and heart disease.

3. Immune System Support

Compounds like carotenoids and glucosinolates enhance immune function by supporting white blood cells and promoting detoxification pathways.

4. Heart Health

Phytonutrients like resveratrol and anthocyanins help lower blood pressure, reduce bad cholesterol levels, and improve arterial health, reducing the risk of heart disease.

5. Cancer Prevention

Certain phytonutrients, like sulforaphane from cruciferous vegetables, have shown promise in cancer prevention. They work by neutralizing carcinogens and promoting the repair of damaged DNA.

6. Enhanced Gut Health

Polyphenols support the growth of beneficial gut bacteria, contributing to improved digestion, reduced inflammation, and better overall health.

Incorporating Phytonutrients into Your Diet

To reap the benefits of phytonutrients, include a variety of colorful fruits, vegetables, legumes, and whole grains in your diet. For example:

- Add leafy greens like spinach and kale to your meals for carotenoids and glucosinolates.
- Snack on berries or nuts for a rich source of polyphenols.
- Incorporate spices like turmeric, rich in curcumin, for added anti-inflammatory benefits.

By diversifying your plant-based food intake, you can ensure an abundant supply of these powerful compounds, supporting long-term health and vitality.

Trendy diets that emphasize extreme imbalances in macronutrient intake, such as high-fat, high-protein, or low-carbohydrate diets, do not support the body's fundamental needs. The body requires a balance of carbohydrates, proteins, and fats to function optimally. Each macronutrient plays a distinct and irreplaceable role in maintaining health. Carbohydrates are the body's primary energy source, fueling the brain, muscles, and vital organs. Proteins are essential for tissue repair, enzyme production, and immune system support. Fats play a crucial role in maintaining cell membrane integrity, hormone synthesis, and the absorption of fat-soluble vitamins (A, D, E, and K).

In addition to macronutrients, the body requires phytonutrients, natural compounds found in plant-based foods that offer antioxidant, anti-inflammatory, and immune-boosting benefits. These compounds, including flavonoids, carotenoids, and polyphenols, play a critical role in protecting against chronic diseases, supporting cellular health, and enhancing metabolic processes. Eliminating or drastically reducing any one macronutrient or neglecting phytonutrients can disrupt these vital processes, leading to metabolic imbalances, nutrient deficiencies, and long-term health risks. While short-term results from such diets may seem appealing, they often come at the expense of overall well-being. A balanced approach that includes appropriate amounts of all three macronutrients, along with phytonutrient-rich foods, is scientifically proven to be the most sustainable and health supportive method for meeting the body's complex physiological needs. This approach ensures comprehensive nourishment for optimal health and long-term well-being.

The Benefits of Fasting

Intermittent Fasting: Health Benefits and Effects on the Body

Intermittent fasting is an integral part of the ASTR Diet, strategically combining fasting periods with an intentional anti-inflammatory approach to nutrition. This combination supports the body's natural healing processes and promotes long-term health. Rather than emphasizing specific food choices during fasting, this method focuses on timing meals to optimize the body's natural healing processes. Popular approaches include the 16:8 method, which involves 16 hours of fasting followed by an 8-hour eating window, and alternate-day fasting.

The ASTR Diet enhances the efficacy of intermittent fasting by emphasizing clean, nutrient-dense, and anti-inflammatory foods during eating periods. This approach maximizes the benefits of fasting, such as improved metabolic health, weight management, and cellular repair. It also prevents setbacks that occur when fasting is broken with inflammatory foods. Together, intermittent fasting and the ASTR Diet create a powerful synergy that supports overall well-being and promotes the body's natural ability to heal.

1. Supports Weight Loss

Intermittent fasting (IF) is an effective method for weight loss as it naturally reduces calorie intake by limiting the eating window. This approach encourages the body to use stored fat for energy during fasting periods, promoting fat burning and weight reduction. A 2020 study published in *Obesity Reviews* found that intermittent fasting results in similar or even greater weight loss compared to traditional calorie-restricted diets. This highlights its effectiveness as a sustainable strategy for weight management.

2. Improves Blood Sugar Control

Intermittent fasting helps regulate blood sugar by lowering insulin levels and improving insulin sensitivity. By limiting frequent glucose spikes, fasting stabilizes blood sugar levels, reducing the risk of insulin resistance and type 2 diabetes. A study published in *Diabetologia* (2014) demonstrated a 3–6% improvement in insulin sensitivity among overweight adults practicing intermittent fasting. This highlights intermittent fasting as a powerful tool for blood sugar management.

3. Reduces Inflammation

Autophagy is a natural, highly regulated cellular process in which the body degrades and recycles damaged or unnecessary cellular components. The term "autophagy" is derived from the Greek words "auto" (self) and "phagy" (eating), meaning "self-eating." This process plays a critical role in maintaining cellular health and homeostasis by eliminating dysfunctional proteins, organelles, and other cellular debris. Autophagy functions like a cellular vacuum, sweeping through cells to remove and dispose of harmful or wasteful components. This process helps ensure that the internal environment remains efficient and functional. By clearing out cellular "clutter," autophagy helps the body optimize energy use, prevent the buildup of toxins, and support overall health and longevity.

Intermittent fasting reduces inflammation by decreasing markers like C-reactive protein and promoting autophagy, the body's natural process for repairing and regenerating cells. This dual action helps combat oxidative stress and chronic inflammation, which are linked to various diseases. Research published in *Cell Metabolism* (2016) highlighted fasting's role in lowering inflammation and enhancing cellular health, contributing to long-term wellness.

4. Enhances Heart Health

Intermittent fasting supports cardiovascular health by reducing LDL cholesterol, triglycerides, and blood pressure. It also improves arterial function, lowering the risk of heart disease. A study published in *The American Journal of Clinical Nutrition* (2015) found that intermittent fasting significantly reduces heart disease risk factors. This makes it a heart-healthy practice with potential long-term benefits.

5. Boosts Brain Function

Intermittent fasting boosts brain health by increasing the production of brain-derived neurotrophic factor (BDNF). This protein plays a key role in supporting memory, learning, and cognitive function. Fasting also promotes autophagy in brain cells, reducing the risk of neurodegenerative diseases such as Alzheimer's and Parkinson's. Animal studies published in *The Journal of Neuroscience* (2013) show that intermittent fasting protects the brain against oxidative stress and age-related decline.

6. Promotes Longevity

Intermittent fasting has been linked to increased lifespan due to its ability to reduce oxidative stress, inflammation, and cellular damage. By enhancing autophagy and improving cellular resilience, fasting supports healthier aging. A 2019 review in *Nature Aging* found that intermittent fasting significantly increased lifespan in animal models and showed promising longevity benefits for humans.

7. Hormonal Changes

Intermittent fasting triggers beneficial hormonal changes that enhance metabolism and fat burning. Insulin levels decrease during fasting, encouraging the body to use stored fat as an energy source. Additionally, intermittent fasting increases human growth hormone (HGH) levels, which helps promote muscle preservation and boosts overall fat metabolism. This makes fasting a highly efficient tool for optimizing metabolic function.

8. Cellular Repair and Autophagy

During fasting, the body activates autophagy, a process where cells remove damaged components and regenerate. This mechanism protects against chronic diseases, supports cellular health, and slows aging. By improving cellular repair, intermittent fasting enhances resilience and reduces the risk of degenerative conditions.

9. Fat Burning and Ketosis

Intermittent fasting encourages fat burning by depleting glycogen stores after 8–12 hours of fasting. Once glycogen is used up, the body switches to ketosis, where fat becomes the primary energy source. This metabolic shift not only promotes efficient fat loss but also improves energy utilization and metabolic health.

10. Improved Gut Health

Fasting gives the digestive system a much-needed break, reducing gut inflammation and promoting healthier gut microbiota. By giving the gut time to rest and repair, intermittent fasting may enhance microbiome diversity and overall digestive health. This can lead to better nutrient absorption and reduced digestive discomfort.

Cautions and Considerations

While intermittent fasting offers numerous health benefits, it may not be appropriate for everyone and requires careful evaluation. Specific groups, including pregnant or breastfeeding women, individuals with a history of eating disorders, and those with certain medical conditions such as diabetes (without proper medical supervision), are advised to avoid intermittent fasting. It is important for these individuals to consult with a healthcare provider before making any dietary changes.

Consulting a clinical nutritionist is essential before starting any fasting regimen, especially for individuals with underlying health conditions, to ensure it is safe and suitable. Additionally, working with a well-trained clinical nutritionist can provide personalized guidance and support, helping to safely implement fasting while optimizing its benefits for overall health.

During the adjustment period, some individuals may experience common side effects such as hunger, fatigue, irritability, or difficulty concentrating. Additionally, there's a risk of overeating during eating windows if mindful eating practices are not followed. To minimize these challenges, starting gradually and building a sustainable routine is key.

4. Practical Tips for Intermittent Fasting

- **Start Gradually:** Begin with a 12:12 fasting-to-eating ratio and work up to longer fasting periods.
- **Stay Hydrated:** Drink water and herbal teas during fasting periods.
- **Focus on Nutrient-Dense Meals:** Prioritize proteins, healthy fats, and whole carbs during eating windows.
- **Plan Your Fasting Schedule:** Align fasting periods with your daily routine for consistency.

Female Fasting Protocol

Women who experience regular menstrual cycles should follow a fasting protocol tailored to their unique hormonal needs to avoid disruptions to period consistency. The female body is highly sensitive to changes in calorie intake and fasting patterns, which can impact hormonal balance. A female-specific fasting protocol typically involves shorter fasting windows, such as 12-14 hours, rather than prolonged fasting periods. This approach is especially important during the luteal phase of the menstrual cycle, when the body requires more energy.

Additionally, consuming nutrient-dense, balanced meals that include healthy fats, proteins, and complex carbohydrates during eating windows supports hormonal health. By aligning fasting practices with their menstrual cycles and prioritizing nourishment, women can enjoy the benefits of intermittent fasting without compromising their period regularity.

- Days 1–10 of the cycle (Day 1 is the first day of full menstrual flow): Any fasting protocol is allowed.

- Days 11–15 of the cycle: Limit fasting to no more than 15 hours.
- Days 16–19 of the cycle: Any fasting protocol is allowed.
- Days 20–28 of the cycle: Avoid fasting altogether.

Why You Should Time Your Last Meal Before Bed

Eating too close to bedtime can harm digestion and overall health, making it essential to allow 4-5 hours between your last meal and sleep. Eating just before lying down causes your body to prioritize digestion over rest and recovery. This can lead to issues such as acid reflux, indigestion, and poor sleep quality. Late-night eating can also disrupt your metabolism, increasing the risk of weight gain and higher blood sugar levels. Leaving a 4-5 hour gap ensures your body has enough time to properly digest food, promoting better sleep, healthier metabolism, and overall wellness. This approach aligns with your body's natural rhythms, allowing it to focus on restoration and healing during sleep rather than expending energy on digestion. Intermittent fasting is a powerful tool for optimizing health and supporting the body's recovery processes.

The Misconceptions About Intermittent Fasting

Intermittent fasting is widely regarded for its potential health benefits, including weight loss, improved metabolism, and cellular detoxification. However, a common misconception is that fasting alone guarantees these outcomes. The truth is that what you consume during your eating windows is just as critical as the fasting period itself. Breaking a fast with inflammatory foods, such as refined carbohydrates, processed snacks, or foods high in pesticides, can undermine the benefits of fasting. It can disrupt the body's recovery and negate the positive effects of the fasting period. For example, consuming sugary pastries or processed fast food after fasting can lead to blood sugar spikes, increased inflammation, and disrupted metabolism. Similarly, foods high in unhealthy fats, artificial additives or chemicals such as pesticide-laden produce or trans-fat-rich fried foods can harm the body. These foods contribute to chronic inflammation and oxidative stress, negatively impacting overall health.

To truly reap the benefits of intermittent fasting, it is essential to focus on nutrient-dense, anti-inflammatory foods during eating windows. These include whole grains, organic fruits and vegetables, proteins, and healthy fats such as avocados, nuts, and olive oil. For instance, breaking a fast with a balanced meal like grilled salmon, quinoa, and steamed broccoli supports detoxification, stabilizes blood sugar, and nourishes the body. This combination provides essential nutrients while promoting overall health. On the other hand, inflammatory food choices can negate the positive effects of fasting, leaving individuals feeling sluggish. These choices can also potentially lead to weight gain instead of weight loss. Ultimately, intermittent fasting is not just about timing; it's about aligning your dietary choices with the body's natural healing processes for sustainable health benefits.

Hydration for Life, Tea for Health

Benefits of Water and Its Role in the Body

Water is essential for life and plays a critical role in maintaining the body's physiological processes. The human body is made up of approximately 50–70% water, varying by age, gender, and body composition.

1. Water Percentage in the Body

Newborns: ~75% water.
Adults: ~50–70% water.
Lean Tissue (Muscle): ~75% water.
Fat Tissue: ~10–15% water.
Older Adults: ~50% water (lower due to decreased muscle mass).

2. Benefits of Water

Water serves as the foundation for various functions in the body. Here's why it's crucial:

A. Hydration and Temperature Regulation

Water plays a critical function in maintaining body temperature, primarily through sweating and respiration. These processes help the body regulate heat and prevent overheating, especially during exercise or in hot environments. By releasing sweat, which evaporates to cool the skin, and through respiratory heat exchange, water helps maintain the body's optimal temperature. This process is crucial for ensuring proper physiological functioning.

B. Cellular Function

Water is essential for maintaining the structure of cells and supporting their function as a building block of life. Water facilitates essential chemical reactions within cells and ensures the transport of nutrients and waste in and out of them. This is crucial for maintaining proper cellular function. Without adequate water, cells cannot maintain their structure, and critical biological processes are disrupted, highlighting water's fundamental role in sustaining life.

C. Blood Circulation

Water plays a vital role in blood circulation, as it constitutes approximately 90% of blood plasma. This high water content is essential for the efficient transport of oxygen, nutrients, and other vital substances throughout the body. By ensuring that nutrients are delivered to tissues effectively, water supports the body's overall function and health. Proper hydration is crucial for maintaining this process, as even mild dehydration can hinder the flow of nutrients and oxygen, leading to reduced energy levels and impaired bodily functions.

D. Joint and Tissue Lubrication

Water is essential for joint and tissue lubrication, playing a key role in maintaining the smooth functioning of various bodily systems. It forms a significant component of synovial fluid, which lubricates joints and reduces friction during movement. This lubrication ensures smooth and pain-free motion while protecting joint structures from wear and tear. Additionally, water provides moisture to the eyes and mucous membranes, maintaining their proper function and comfort. Adequate hydration is crucial for preserving these protective mechanisms and promoting overall mobility and well-being.

E. Waste Removal

Water plays a crucial role in waste removal by supporting kidney function. It helps flush out toxins and waste products from the body through urine, ensuring that harmful substances are efficiently eliminated. Proper hydration is crucial to prevent the buildup of waste in the body. Without adequate water intake, conditions such as kidney stones and urinary tract infections can develop. By maintaining adequate water intake, the kidneys can function optimally, promoting overall health and reducing the risk of complications associated with inadequate waste removal.

F. Digestion and Nutrient Absorption

Water is essential for digestion and nutrient absorption, playing a key role in breaking down food and facilitating the body's ability to utilize nutrients. It aids in saliva production, which is the first step in digestion, helping to moisten and break down food for easier swallowing and processing. Additionally, water dissolves minerals and nutrients, making them more readily absorbable in the digestive tract. Proper hydration ensures that these processes function efficiently, supporting overall health and optimal nutrient uptake.

G. Brain Function

Water is essential for maintaining optimal brain function, as it helps regulate cognitive processes and prevent symptoms such as fatigue and confusion. Proper hydration ensures that the brain operates efficiently, supporting memory, concentration, and overall mental clarity. Even mild dehydration can significantly impair these functions, leading to reduced focus and cognitive performance. By staying adequately hydrated, individuals can enhance their brain's ability to process information and perform at its best.

H. Energy Production

Water is vital for energy production, as it facilitates key metabolic reactions, including the conversion of food into usable energy. Proper hydration ensures that these processes occur efficiently, supporting the body's ability to maintain physical and mental performance. When the body is dehydrated, metabolism slows, leading to decreased energy levels and reduced physical performance. Staying adequately hydrated is essential for sustaining energy, optimizing metabolic function, and enhancing overall vitality.

I. Skin Health

Water is essential for maintaining skin health by keeping it hydrated and preserving its elasticity. Proper hydration helps prevent dryness, keeping the skin smooth and supple. Additionally, water plays a critical role in supporting wound healing by promoting cell regeneration and maintaining the skin's protective barrier. Staying adequately hydrated enhances skin appearance and function, contributing to overall health and resilience.

Water is vital for nearly every bodily function, from cellular health to waste removal and cognitive performance. Ensuring adequate hydration supports overall health and prevents dehydration-related complications. Regular water intake, adjusted for activity levels and environmental conditions, is key to maintaining balance in the body.

Hidden Dangers in Tap Water

The quality of tap water varies widely across regions and is influenced by factors such as industrial activities, agricultural runoff, and aging infrastructure. Common contaminants in tap water may include heavy metals, per- and polyfluoroalkyl substances (PFAS), microorganisms, pharmaceutical residues, pesticides, and disinfection byproducts. These substances can pose potential health risks, underscoring the importance of regular water quality assessments and appropriate filtration methods to ensure safe consumption.

Common Contaminants in Tap Water

Heavy Metals: Lead and arsenic are prevalent in some water supplies, often due to corroding pipes or natural deposits. Exposure to these metals can lead to serious health issues, including neurological damage and increased cancer risk.

Per- and Polyfluoroalkyl Substances (PFAS): Often called "forever chemicals" due to their persistence in the environment originate from a variety of industrial and consumer sources. They are widely used in non-stick cookware, waterproof clothing, stain-resistant fabrics, food packaging, and firefighting foams, as well as in certain cleaning agents, cosmetics, and industrial processes. PFAS can contaminate water supplies, soil, and air through industrial discharge, agricultural runoff from PFAS-containing biosolids, and the use of firefighting foams. These contaminants can persist in the environment, posing long-term health risks. Once released, these chemicals persist in the environment, leaching into groundwater, accumulating in soil, and spreading through atmospheric deposition. Human exposure to PFAS occurs mainly through drinking contaminated water, consuming fish or animals exposed to these chemicals, and contact with PFAS-treated products. This underscores the need for stringent controls and effective remediation efforts to reduce exposure and protect public health.

A U.S. Geological Survey study estimated that at least 45% of the nation's tap water contains one or more types of PFAS. These chemicals are linked to various health problems, including immune system effects and certain cancers.

Microorganisms: Bacteria, viruses, and parasites can contaminate water sources, leading to illnesses such as gastrointestinal infections. While treatment processes aim to eliminate these pathogens, breaches in the system can result in contamination.

Disinfection Byproducts: Chemicals like trihalomethanes form when disinfectants used in water treatment react with natural organic matter. Long-term exposure to these byproducts has been associated with liver, kidney, or central nervous system problems, and an increased risk of cancer.

Water Contamination Studies

Recent studies have highlighted various contaminants present in tap water, raising concerns about public health. Here are some key findings:

PFAS Contamination: A U.S. Geological Survey study found that at least 45% of the nation's tap water contains one or more types of per- and polyfluoroalkyl substances (PFAS), often referred to as "forever chemicals" due to their persistence in the environment.

Fluoride Levels and Cognitive Effects: Research indicates a statistically significant correlation between higher levels of fluoride in drinking water and lower IQ levels in children. There is no need to add fluoride to water supplies.

Microplastics in Tap Water: Studies have detected synthetic polymers, commonly known as microplastics, in tap water, beer, and sea salt. This raises concerns about the potential health implications of ingesting these particles.

Unregulated 'Forever Chemicals' in Europe: Investigations have revealed the presence of trifluoroacetic acid (TFA), an unmonitored PFAS, in the drinking water of several European cities, including Paris. This contamination is primarily due to the degradation of pesticides and fluorinated gases.

Chlorination Byproducts: A previously unknown chemical, chloronitramide anion, has been identified in chloramine-treated drinking water in the U.S. This stable byproduct forms from the decomposition of chloramine, a disinfectant used in water treatment. Its health impacts are currently under investigation.

These findings underscore the importance of regular monitoring and updating water treatment practices to address emerging contaminants and ensure the safety of public drinking water supplies.

Health Implications:

Exposure to water contaminants, even in small amounts, can lead to cumulative health risks over time. For example, PFAS (per- and polyfluoroalkyl substances) have been associated with immune system suppression, which can weaken the body's ability to respond to illnesses. Additionally, heavy metals like lead are well-known for their harmful effects on children's development, contributing to learning disabilities, behavioral issues, and long-term cognitive impairments. Addressing water contamination is essential to safeguarding public health, particularly in vulnerable populations.

Regional Variations:

Studies have shown that tap water contamination is not uniformly distributed. Urban areas may experience different types of pollutants compared to rural regions, often due to industrial discharges and higher population densities. For example, PFAS contamination has been detected in various U.S. cities, with exposure disproportionately affecting communities of color.

Types of Water Filters and What They Remove

Water filters come in various types, each designed to remove specific contaminants from water. Here's an overview of the common types, their capabilities, and effectiveness:

Activated carbon filters work by adsorbing contaminants onto a porous carbon surface, effectively removing chlorine (up to 99%), sediment, particulates, volatile organic compounds (VOCs), some pesticides, herbicides, and odors. This process improves the taste and quality of the water. However, they are less effective at removing heavy metals, nitrates, or bacteria, with an effectiveness range of 90-99% for targeted chemicals.

Reverse Osmosis (RO) Systems utilize a semipermeable membrane to filter out heavy metals like lead, arsenic, and mercury, as well as nitrates, fluoride, bacteria, viruses, and up to 99% of dissolved salts and minerals.

Distillation Units purify water by boiling it to create steam and then condensing it back into liquid form. This process effectively removes heavy metals, most bacteria and viruses, and salts, achieving 99% effectiveness for inorganic contaminants and microbes. However, they are ineffective against VOCs and some pesticides, as these evaporate along with the water.

UV (Ultraviolet) Filters use UV light to destroy the DNA of bacteria, viruses, and other pathogens, eliminating up to 99.9% of microbial threats. However, they do not remove chemicals, heavy metals, or particulates, making them primarily suitable for microbial disinfection.

Ceramic Filters rely on tiny pores in ceramic material to trap particulates and microorganisms, effectively removing sediment, bacteria, and protozoa. While they are 80-99% effective against microbes and particulates, they do not filter out chemicals or heavy metals.

Ion exchange filters replace undesirable ions like calcium and magnesium with less harmful ones such as sodium or potassium. This process effectively addresses hard water minerals and can also remove some heavy metals. However, they are ineffective against bacteria, viruses, and organic contaminants, with a removal efficiency of 90-95% for hardness and metals.

Alkaline Water Filters enhance water pH by adding minerals like calcium and magnesium. While they can remove chlorine and some heavy metals, their primary function is pH adjustment, offering limited purification capabilities (10-50% for contaminants).

Alkaline water filters, while popular for their ability to adjust water pH, contribute only minimally to the body's mineral intake due to the trace amounts of minerals they provide. Although these filters may slightly enhance hydration and neutralize acidity, they should not be relied upon as a primary source of essential nutrients. The most effective and natural way to meet the body's mineral requirements is through a diet rich in nuts, seeds, fruits, and vegetables. These foods offer an abundant and bioavailable supply of vital minerals, such as potassium, magnesium, and calcium, along with antioxidants and phytonutrients that support overall health. Incorporating a variety of fresh, nutrient-dense whole foods ensures the body receives the minerals it needs far more effectively than relying on filtered water.

Gravity-Fed Filters pass water through multiple filtration stages using gravity, removing sediments, microbial pathogens (in advanced models), and chemicals like chlorine. Their effectiveness varies widely based on the system, ranging from 80-99% depending on the contaminants and filter design.

Water Filter Comparison

Filter Type	Microbes	Chemicals	Heavy Metals	Sediments	Hardness
Activated Carbon	No	Yes	Partial	Yes	No
Reverse Osmosis	Yes	Yes	Yes	Yes	Yes
Distillation	Yes	Partial	Yes	Yes	No
UV Filters	Yes	No	No	No	No
Ceramic Filters	Partial	No	No	Yes	No
Ion Exchange	No	No	Partial	No	Yes
Alkaline Filters	No	Partial	Partial	No	No
Gravity-Fed	Partial	Partial	Partial	Yes	No

Best Water Filter

Reverse osmosis (RO) is widely regarded as the best option for water filtration due to its unparalleled effectiveness in removing a broad range of contaminants. Using a semipermeable membrane, RO systems can eliminate up to 99% of dissolved salts, heavy metals (such as lead, arsenic, and mercury), nitrates, fluoride, and even bacteria and viruses.

This comprehensive filtration process ensures the highest level of water purity, making it ideal for households and individuals concerned about health and safety.

Unlike other filtration methods that may target specific contaminants, RO provides an all-encompassing solution, addressing both organic and inorganic impurities. While it does have limitations, such as water wastage during the purification process, advances in technology have minimized these drawbacks. For those seeking the cleanest, safest drinking water, reverse osmosis remains the gold standard. There are many excellent countertop reverse osmosis systems available online that do not require plumbing.

Herbal Teas and Their Health Benefits

Herbal teas are made from various parts of plants, including leaves, flowers, seeds, and roots. They offer numerous health benefits due to their unique compositions. Below is a detailed list:

1. Green Tea

- **Rich in Antioxidants:**
  Green tea contains catechins, especially EGCG (epigallocatechin gallate), which combat free radicals, reduce oxidative stress, and promote overall health.

- **Weight Loss and Metabolism:**
  Green tea boosts metabolism and supports fat oxidation, aiding in weight management. Studies show green tea extract can enhance fat burning by up to 17% during exercise.

- **Heart Health:**
  Green tea lowers LDL cholesterol and improves artery function, significantly reducing the risk of cardiovascular disease. Research indicates green tea drinkers have a 31% lower risk of heart disease.

- **Brain Health:**
  The combination of EGCG and caffeine in green tea enhances memory, focus, and brain function. It may also reduce the risk of neurodegenerative diseases such as Alzheimer's and Parkinson's.

- **Diabetes Management:**
  Green tea improves insulin sensitivity and lowers blood sugar levels. Studies suggest regular consumption may reduce the risk of type 2 diabetes by 33%.

- **Anti-Cancer Properties:**
  EGCG in green tea has been shown to inhibit cancer cell growth and reduce the risk of various cancers, including breast, prostate, and colorectal cancers.

2. Black Tea

Black tea is rich in flavonoids, which improve heart health by enhancing blood vessel function and lowering blood pressure. Regular consumption is linked to a 10% reduction in the risk of cardiovascular disease, as supported by studies.

- **Antioxidant Properties:**
  Black tea contains powerful polyphenols, including theaflavins and thearubigins, which protect cells from oxidative damage and help reduce inflammation throughout the body.

- **Digestive Health:**
  The tannins in black tea have anti-inflammatory effects that support gut health and may improve the diversity of gut microbiota, contributing to a healthy digestive system.

- **Mental Alertness:**
  With caffeine and L-theanine, black tea enhances focus and reduces

fatigue. It improves reaction times and cognitive performance, making it an excellent choice for maintaining mental alertness.

- **Cancer Prevention:**
  Antioxidants in black tea may help lower the risk of certain cancers, particularly those affecting the skin, lungs, and breasts. They do so by combating oxidative stress and inhibiting cancer cell growth.

3. Chamomile Tea

Chamomile tea is well-known for its calming properties, making it an excellent choice for reducing stress and anxiety. It also improves sleep quality and soothes digestive issues such as bloating and gas. Additionally, its anti-inflammatory properties can help relieve menstrual cramps, making it a versatile herbal remedy.

4. Peppermint Tea

Peppermint tea is a refreshing option that aids digestion and relieves bloating. It is also known for soothing headaches and migraines, freshening breath, and reducing nausea. Furthermore, it may improve focus, making it a revitalizing choice for mental clarity.

5. Ginger Tea

Ginger tea is highly effective for reducing nausea caused by motion sickness or morning sickness. Its anti-inflammatory properties help alleviate arthritis pain, while it also boosts immune function and aids digestion by reducing bloating.

6. Hibiscus Tea

Hibiscus tea is celebrated for its ability to lower blood pressure and promote heart health due to its rich antioxidant content. It supports liver health and may assist with weight management, making it a nutritious and tangy option.

7. Rooibos Tea

Rooibos tea is caffeine-free and rich in antioxidants, supporting skin health and lowering blood pressure. It may also help reduce allergy symptoms, making it a soothing and relaxing herbal tea choice.

8. Lemon Balm Tea

Lemon balm tea reduces stress and promotes relaxation, making it a great choice for unwinding. It also improves mood, cognitive function, and digestion, while helping with mild insomnia and anxiety.

9. Echinacea Tea

Echinacea tea is widely used to boost the immune system and reduce the severity and duration of colds. Its anti-inflammatory and antioxidant properties also contribute to overall health and wellness.

10. Lavender Tea

Lavender tea is an excellent choice for relaxation and better sleep. It reduces stress and anxiety, soothes headaches, and supports digestive health, offering a gentle way to unwind.

11. Turmeric Tea

Turmeric tea is packed with anti-inflammatory and antioxidant properties, making it beneficial for reducing arthritis pain and supporting liver detoxification. It also boosts immune function, adding to its wide-ranging health benefits.

12. Dandelion Tea

Dandelion tea supports liver health and detoxification while acting as a natural diuretic to reduce water retention. It may also help with weight management and is rich in vitamins and minerals that support overall well-being.

13. Fenugreek Tea

Fenugreek tea aids digestion, reduces bloating, and supports lactation in breastfeeding mothers. It may also help lower blood sugar levels and has anti-inflammatory properties.

14. Fennel Tea

Fennel tea is excellent for relieving bloating, gas, and indigestion. It supports lactation in breastfeeding mothers, promotes skin health with its antioxidants, and helps regulate appetite for better dietary balance.

15. Licorice Root Tea

Licorice root tea is soothing for sore throats and coughs, making it ideal for cold relief. It also improves digestive health, reduces inflammation, and supports adrenal gland health to manage stress effectively.

15. Cinnamon Tea

Cinnamon tea helps stabilize blood sugar levels and offers anti-inflammatory and antimicrobial benefits. It improves circulation and may assist with weight management, making it both flavorful and functional.

16. Sage Tea

Sage tea supports cognitive health and memory, making it beneficial for brain function. It also helps reduce menopausal symptoms, aids digestion, and is rich in antioxidants for overall wellness.

17. Thyme Tea

Thyme tea is known for fighting respiratory infections and soothing coughs. Its antibacterial and antifungal properties support immune health, while it also aids digestion and provides antioxidant protection.

18. Nettle Tea

Nettle tea is packed with essential vitamins and minerals like iron, calcium, and magnesium, supporting overall health. It reduces inflammation, helps with seasonal allergies, and supports kidney and urinary health.

19. Rosehip Tea

Rosehip tea is rich in vitamin C, boosting immune health and promoting skin vitality. Its anti-inflammatory properties can reduce joint pain, and it also supports heart health, making it a nutritious choice.

20. Valerian Root Tea

Valerian root tea is a natural remedy for relaxation and better sleep. It reduces stress and anxiety, soothes muscle tension, and is highly effective for managing insomnia.

21. Holy Basil (Tulsi) Tea

Holy basil tea is a powerful adaptogen that reduces stress and supports adrenal health. It boosts immune function, regulates blood sugar, and provides anti-inflammatory and antioxidant benefits.

22. Parsley Tea

Parsley tea acts as a natural diuretic, reducing water retention and supporting kidney and urinary health. It is rich in vitamin K, which promotes bone health, and contains antioxidants that enhance overall wellness.

Regardless of the type, teas offer shared benefits such as boosting the immune system, promoting hydration, supporting oral health, and relieving stress. Incorporating a variety of teas into your daily routine provides a natural, enjoyable way to enhance overall well-being and address specific health needs.

Snack Smart

Healthy Snacks and Their Benefits

Healthy snacks play a crucial role in the ASTR diet by maintaining energy levels, curbing hunger, and providing essential nutrients between meals. Choosing nutrient-dense options like nuts, seeds, fresh fruits, and vegetables aligns with the ASTR diet's principles of being anti-inflammatory, sustainable, toxin-free, and restorative. These snacks not only support overall health but also help prevent overeating by promoting satiety and stabilizing blood sugar levels. Whether it's a handful of almonds, a mix of sunflower and chia seeds, crisp apple slices, or crunchy carrot sticks, these simple and wholesome choices keep you energized throughout the day. They align with the ASTR diet's focus on clean, balanced nutrition. Let's explore these options in detail.

1. Nuts

Nuts are a convenient, portable, and nutrient-dense snack packed with healthy fats, protein, and essential vitamins. Examples: Almonds, walnuts, cashews, pistachios, pecans, hazelnuts.

Nutritional Benefits:

Nuts offer a wide range of nutritional benefits that make them an excellent addition to a healthy diet. For heart health, nuts are rich in monounsaturated and polyunsaturated fats, which help lower LDL cholesterol and support overall cardiovascular function. They are also loaded with antioxidants like vitamin E and polyphenols, which combat inflammation and protect the heart. Nuts are a great source of plant-based protein, aiding in muscle repair and providing a steady release of energy to prevent crashes. For brain health, walnuts stand out as they are high in omega-3 fatty acids, which enhance cognitive function and may protect against neurodegenerative diseases. Additionally, nuts are rich in key micronutrients like magnesium, which supports muscle relaxation and energy production, and selenium, which boosts immunity and promotes thyroid function. These nutrients contribute to overall health and well-being. This combination of nutrients makes nuts a powerhouse for overall health and well-being.

Portion Tip:

Stick to a handful (about 1 ounce) to avoid overconsumption, as nuts are calorie-dense.

2. Seeds

Seeds are small but mighty nutritional powerhouses, offering fiber, protein, and healthy fats. Examples: Chia seeds, flaxseeds, sunflower seeds, pumpkin seeds, sesame seeds.

Nutritional Benefits:

Seeds are a nutritional powerhouse, offering a variety of health benefits, particularly for digestive health. They are rich in both soluble and insoluble fiber, which promote gut health, support healthy digestion, and ensure regular bowel movements. Seeds like flaxseeds and chia seeds are also abundant in omega-3 fatty acids, which reduce inflammation and support heart health. Additionally, they are packed with essential micronutrients such as zinc, which boosts immunity and aids in wound healing, and magnesium, which supports muscle function and energy metabolism. These nutrients play vital roles in maintaining overall health. Incorporating seeds into your diet is an easy way to enhance overall health and nutrition.

Special Note on Chia Seeds: Form a gel-like consistency when soaked, making them excellent for hydration and digestion.

3. Fresh Fruits

Fresh fruits are nature's sweet, hydrating snacks that deliver essential vitamins, fiber, and antioxidants. Examples: Apples, bananas, oranges, berries (strawberries, blueberries, raspberries), watermelon, kiwi, mangos.

Nutritional Benefits:

Fruits are a nutrient-dense and versatile food group packed with numerous health benefits. They are rich in antioxidants, with berries being particularly high in anthocyanins, which protect cells from damage and support heart health. Fruits provide natural sugars, offering a quick energy boost without added sugars, making them ideal for pre- or post-workout snacks. Many fruits, like watermelon and oranges, are also water-rich, helping to maintain hydration levels. Additionally, fruits such as apples and pears are excellent sources of soluble fiber, like pectin, which supports gut health and helps regulate blood sugar levels. Fruits are rich in essential vitamins and minerals. For example, vitamin C from citrus fruits boosts immunity and promotes skin health, while potassium from bananas helps regulate blood pressure. Including a variety of fruits in your diet is an easy and delicious way to support overall health.

3. Fresh Vegetables

Vegetables make excellent snacks that are both healthy and satisfying. Crunchy options like carrot sticks, cucumber slices, celery sticks, and bell pepper strips are easy to prepare and enjoy raw. Cherry tomatoes and sugar snap peas are sweet and flavorful, making them appealing for quick bites. For added variety, vegetables like broccoli florets, cauliflower, or zucchini slices can be paired with hummus, guacamole, or a yogurt-based dip. These options are not only convenient but also versatile, making them ideal for on-the-go snacking or as part of a healthy lunchbox.

Nutritional Benefits:

Snacking on vegetables offers numerous health benefits. They are naturally low in calories but rich in fiber, which helps promote satiety and supports digestive health. Vegetables are rich in essential vitamins and minerals like vitamin C, potassium, and folate. These nutrients help boost immunity, regulate blood pressure, and support overall well-being. Additionally, their high water content aids hydration and keeps you feeling refreshed. Unlike processed snacks, vegetables are free of added sugars and unhealthy fats, making them a nutrient-dense choice that supports long-term health and weight management. Incorporating vegetables as snacks is an easy way to meet daily recommended servings and improve overall nutrition.

3 Steps to Transform Your Health

Transforming your health doesn't have to feel overwhelming. In just three simple steps, you can make significant progress: remove unhealthy food from your home, create a thoughtful shopping list, and purchase the right ingredients. Preparation is key to success. As Benjamin Franklin said, "Failing to plan is planning to fail." With the ASTR diet, careful planning and intentional execution will guide you toward lasting health and healing.

Step 1: Throw Out Bad Food

Begin by clearing out your pantry, refrigerator, and freezer of unhealthy, processed, and toxin-laden foods. **The only effective approach is a cold turkey approach.** Do not postpone or attempt to remove unhealthy items gradually, as this method often fails. Eliminating all "bad foods" at once ensures a clean slate and reduces the temptation to revert to old habits. Remove items that contain artificial additives, trans fats, excessive sugars, and refined carbohydrates. Replace these with fresh, whole, anti-inflammatory ingredients that align with the ASTR diet. This decisive action creates space for nourishing, healing options and sets the stage for success.

Step 2: Create a Shopping List

A well-prepared shopping list is essential for staying on track. Include ingredients that align with the ASTR diet, such as healthy fats (e.g., avocados, nuts, seeds, olive oil), clean proteins (e.g., meats, fish, eggs, plant-based options), and complex carbohydrates (e.g., quinoa, sweet potatoes, whole grains). This ensures you're stocked with the right foods for balanced, nutritious meals. Include anti-inflammatory foods like leafy greens, turmeric, ginger, and berries, while ensuring the ingredients are toxin-free and sustainable. This list will not only guide your shopping trip but also save time and reduce unnecessary purchases.

Step 3: Go Shopping

With your shopping list in hand, visit grocery stores or farmers' markets to stock up on fresh, nutrient-dense foods. Choose organic and locally sourced options when possible to minimize exposure to harmful chemicals and support sustainability. By prioritizing quality ingredients, you're building the foundation for a healthier, more balanced lifestyle.

How to Implement the ASTR Diet

Once you've stocked your kitchen, it's time to integrate the ASTR diet into your daily routine. The key to success lies in planning every aspect of your day around balanced and intentional eating.

1. **Plan Your Day:** Structure your meals and snacks to fit within your lifestyle. Decide on an eating window, especially if incorporating intermittent fasting, and stick to it.
2. **Eating Window:** Implement an eating window that works for you, such as 4-8 hours of eating followed by 16-20 hours of fasting. One of the easiest ways to implement fasting is by eating during typical workday hours, such as 8:00 AM to 5:00 PM or 9:00 AM to 6:00 PM. This promotes metabolic efficiency and supports the body's natural healing processes. Maintain a 4-5-hour gap between your last meal and sleep.
3. **Plan Your Snacks:** Prepare healthy snacks like raw nuts, vegetables, or fruit in advance to avoid reaching for processed options. Snacks should align with the ASTR diet principles.
4. **80%-90% Rule:** Aim to follow the ASTR diet 80% to 90% of the time, allowing for flexibility while maintaining consistent progress. This realistic approach ensures long-term adherence without feeling restrictive.
5. **Eat What You Love for Lasting Success:** The most important part of the ASTR diet is starting with the shopping list and choosing foods you genuinely enjoy eating. This personalized approach ensures that the diet feels sustainable and enjoyable, rather than restrictive or burdensome. When you select foods that you like, you are more likely to remain consistent with the diet, making it easier to stick to long-term. Enjoying what you eat fosters a positive relationship with

food, helping you build healthier habits without feeling deprived. This approach ultimately supports your health and wellness goals, making it easier to maintain long-term.

6. **Cook Once, Eat All Week:** For individuals with a busy schedule, planning and preparing meals in advance can be a game-changer. By dedicating time over the weekend to cook your meals, you can ensure that healthy, home-cooked options are readily available throughout the week. Once prepared, refrigerate the meals in portioned containers to maintain freshness. When it's time to eat, simply reheat them on the stove to preserve their flavor and nutritional value.

I like to prepare my dry breakfast cereal ingredients in advance, mixing them in a sealed container to last for up to two weeks. This simple preparation saves time in the morning, allowing me to quickly scoop out a portion of my breakfast cereal without needing to mix ingredients every day. All that's left to do is add milk and butter, making breakfast both convenient and stress-free. This method ensures I stick to my routine while enjoying a wholesome, ready-to-go meal to start the day. This approach not only saves time during hectic weekdays but also promotes healthier eating habits by reducing reliance on takeout or processed foods.

Final Thoughts

By throwing out bad food with a decisive cold turkey approach, creating a targeted shopping list, and shopping intentionally, you're setting the stage for success. Coupled with thoughtful planning, an intentional eating window, and the 80%-90% rule, the ASTR diet provides a sustainable pathway to transform your health in just 30 days. With preparation and dedication, you can enjoy balanced meals, improved well-being, and a stronger, healthier body.

Addendum

Key Points

ASTR Diet

A - Anti-inflammatory
S - Sustainable
T - Toxin-free
R - Restorative

ASTR Plate: 1/3 Fat, 1/3 Protein, 1/3 Carbohydrates

Water filter: Reverse osmosis 4-5 stages

Snack Smart: fruits, vegetables, nuts and seeds

Dinner: Eat 4-5 hours before sleeping

Fasting: Recommended eating time per day: 4–8 hours. Outside of this window, engage in water and tea fasting

Check the Product's Ethics: cornucopia.org/scorecards

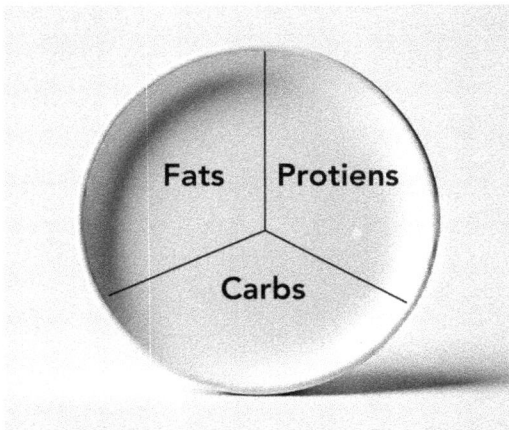

ASTR

Foods To Avoid List

Common Culprits:
- Refined sugar
- Artificial sweeteners
- High fructose corn syrup
- Refined carbs (e.g., candy, desserts)
- Gluten
- Cassava root (tapioca)

Processed and GMO Foods:
- GMO products
- Processed food
- Soy products
- Corn products
- Food additives & colors

Dairy and Beverages:
- Pasteurized dairy products
- Soft drinks (sodas)
- Energy drinks
- Alcohol
- Juices

Fats and Fried Foods:
- Fried foods
- Hydrogenated & trans fats
- Seed oils

Seafood and Nuts:
- Farmed fish
- Peanut products
- Large fish: max 3-4 times/month

ASTR

Short Shopping List

Short Shopping List

Proteins:
- Chicken (free-range)
- Turkey (free-range))
- Beef, lamb, bison, venison (organic, grass-fed)
- Raw whole milk
- Salmon (Alaskan or sockeye)
- Sardine
- Anchovy
- Squid

Fats:
- Avocados
- Nuts and seeds
- Raw cacao butter
- Eggs (organic, free-range, soy, and corn free)
- Organic grass-fed butter and ghee

Whole Foods:
- Quinoa, brown rice, millet, buckwheat and amaranth
- A wide variety of fruits and vegetables
- Mushrooms (Lion's Mane, Shiitake, Oyster, Maitake, etc.)

Fermented Foods:
- Fermented vegetables & pickles
- Kimchi
- Sauerkraut
- Raw whole milk kefir
- Raw cheese
- Kombucha (non-alcoholic)
- Apple cider vinegar with "the mother" (unrefined, unpasteurized)

Oils (with Smoke Points):
- Avocado oil (520°F)
- Coconut oil (350°F)
- Extra virgin olive oil (320°F)

ASTR

Full Shopping List

Fruits
- **Non-GMO & Organic**: Choose non-GMO fruits and prioritize organic options.
- Citrus: Orange, Grapefruit, Tangerines, Lemon, Lime
- Berries: Berries, Cranberries
- Tropical: Mango, Passion fruit, Papaya, Pineapple, Guava
- Common: Banana, Apple, Pears, Peaches, Plums, Rhubarb, Kiwi, Melons
- Dried: Raisins, Dates, Figs
- Exotic: Pomegranates, Tomatoes, Olives

Vegetables
- Broccoli
- Spinach
- Kale
- Carrots
- Cucumber
- Cabbage
- Celery
- Garlic
- Onion
- Potatoes
- Pickles
- Kimchi
- Sauerkraut
- Artichoke
- Bean sprouts
- Bok choy
- Brussels sprouts
- Cauliflower
- Okra
- Radish
- Snow peas
- Zucchini
- Bell peppers

ASTR

Protein
- Legumes (Beans & Lentils)
- Chicken, Turkey (Free-Range))
- Eggs (Organic, Free-Range, Soy- and Corn-Free)
- Beef, Lamb, Bison, Venison (Organic, Grass-fed)
- Wild Fish (e.g., Salmon – Alaskan or sockeye, Sardines, Anchovy, Squid)
- *Large Fish*: Limit consumption to 3–4 times a month

Fats
- Coconut oil
- Grass-fed butter (e.g., Kerrygold)
- Grass-fed ghee
- Extra virgin olive oil
- Avocado oil
- Raw cacao butter

Gluten-Free Grains
- Quinoa
- Brown rice
- Millet
- Buckwheat
- Amaranth

Drinks
- Green/Black tea
- Herbal teas
- Mushroom tea

Spices
- All pure spices
- Himalayan salt

Nuts & Seeds
- Nuts: Brazil nuts, Walnuts, Macadamia nuts, Pistachio, Almonds

ASTR

- Seeds: Chia, Sunflower, Hemp, Flax, Pumpkin

Baking
- Coconut flour
- Brown rice flour
- Almond flour/meal
- Arrowroot flour

Sweeteners
- Unfiltered raw honey
- Coconut sugar
- Date sugar
- Pure maple syrup

Dressings
- Apple cider vinegar
- Lemon/Lime juice
- Balsamic vinegar

ASTR

Recipes

Recipes

1. Dr. Jacobs' Breakfast

Ingredients:

- Chia seeds: 1 tablespoon
- Cocoa powder: 1 teaspoon
- Flaxseeds: 1 tablespoon
- Oatmeal: 1 tablespoon (rolled oats)
- Raisins: 2 tablespoons
- Cold raw milk: ½ cup
- Butter: 3-4 tablespoon (melted)
- Mixed nuts: 2 tablespoons
- Blueberries: 2 tablespoons

Instructions:

1. Mix oatmeal, chia seeds, flaxseeds, cocoa powder, and raisins in a bowl.
2. Pour cold raw milk over the mixture and stir well.
3. Drizzle melted butter over the top and mix gently.
4. Top with blueberries and nuts.
5. Let sit for 5 minutes before eating to allow the oats and chia seeds to soften.

2. Raisin Apple Breakfast Bowl

Ingredients:

- Chia seeds: 2 teaspoons
- Flaxseeds: 1 tablespoon
- Oatmeal: ½ cup (rolled oats)
- Raisins: 1 tablespoon
- Cold raw milk: ½ cup
- Butter: 3-4 tablespoon (softened)
- Mixed nuts: 2 tablespoons (chopped)
- Apple: ½ diced

Instructions:

1. Combine oatmeal, chia seeds, flaxseeds, and raisins in a bowl.
2. Stir in softened butter to coat the dry ingredients.
3. Pour cold raw milk over the mixture and stir well.
4. Add diced apples and mixed nuts on top.
5. Serve immediately for a crunchy and sweet breakfast.

3. Creamy Chocolate Berry Bowl with Strawberries

Ingredients:

- Chia seeds: 1 tablespoon
- Cocoa powder: 1 tablespoon
- Flaxseeds: 1 tablespoon
- Oatmeal: ½ cup (rolled oats)
- Raisins: 1 tablespoon
- Cold raw milk: ½ cup
- Butter: 3 tablespoon (melted)
- Strawberries: ¼ cup (sliced)
- Mixed nuts: 1 tablespoon

Instructions:

1. In a bowl, mix oatmeal, chia seeds, flaxseeds, cocoa powder, and raisins.
2. Pour cold raw milk into the bowl and stir until combined.
3. Drizzle melted butter over the mixture.
4. Top with sliced strawberries and a sprinkle of mixed nuts.
5. Serve immediately.

4. Tropical Nutty Protein Bowl with Mango

Ingredients:

- Chia seeds: 1 tablespoon

- Flaxseeds: 1 tablespoon
- Oatmeal: ½ cup (rolled oats)
- Raisins: 2 tablespoons
- Cold raw milk: ½ cup
- Butter: 3 tablespoon (melted)
- Mixed nuts: 2 tablespoons (chopped)
- Mango: ½ cup (diced)

Instructions:

1. Combine oatmeal, chia seeds, flaxseeds, and raisins in a bowl.
2. Pour cold raw milk over the mixture and stir thoroughly.
3. Drizzle melted butter on top and mix gently.
4. Add diced mango and chopped nuts as a topping.
5. Serve chilled for a refreshing and tropical-flavored bowl.

4. Herb-Crusted Salmon with Quinoa

Ingredients:

- 4 oz grilled salmon
- ½ cup cooked quinoa
- 2 tablespoon avocado oil
- 1 cup steamed broccoli and zucchini
- Garlic powder, dill, lemon zest, and salt
- Fresh lemon juice

Instructions:

1. Season salmon with garlic powder, dill, lemon zest, and salt.
2. Grill or bake salmon until cooked through.
3. Cook quinoa according to package instructions.
4. Steam broccoli and zucchini until tender.
5. Drizzle salmon with avocado oil and squeeze fresh lemon juice before serving.

5. Spiced Chicken and Brown Rice Bowl

Ingredients:

- 4 oz grilled chicken breast (sliced)
- ½ cup cooked brown rice
- 2 tablespoon extra virgin olive oil
- ¼ teaspoon apple cider vinegar
- 1 cup roasted carrots and green beans
- Paprika, cumin, garlic powder, and black pepper
- Chopped parsley

Instructions:

1. Season chicken with paprika, cumin, garlic powder, and black pepper.
2. Grill chicken and slice into strips.
3. Cook brown rice according to package instructions.
4. Roast carrots and green beans until tender.
5. Drizzle olive oil over the chicken and rice.
6. Garnish with parsley before serving.

6. Mediterranean Sardine Plate

Ingredients:

- 1 can sardines (drained)
- ½ cup cooked quinoa
- 2 tablespoon extra virgin olive oil
- 1 cup mixed greens, cherry tomatoes, cucumbers, and red onions
- Oregano, sumac, and sea salt
- Balsamic vinegar

Instructions:

1. Drain sardines and place on a plate.
2. Cook quinoa according to package instructions.
3. Arrange mixed greens, cherry tomatoes, cucumbers, and red onions.
4. Drizzle olive oil and balsamic vinegar over vegetables.
5. Sprinkle with oregano, sumac, and sea salt.
6. Serve sardines alongside quinoa and salad.

7. Garlic Butter Beef Stir-Fry

Ingredients:

- 4 oz thinly sliced grass-fed beef
- ½ cup cooked brown rice
- 2 tablespoon grass-fed butter
- 1 cup sautéed broccoli, bell peppers, and snap peas
- ¼ teaspoon apple cider vinegar
- Garlic, black pepper, and red pepper flakes
- Green onions (for garnish)

Instructions:

1. Pan-sear beef slices until cooked through.
2. Cook brown rice according to package instructions.
3. Sauté broccoli, bell peppers, and snap peas in the same pan.
4. Season vegetables with garlic, black pepper, apple cider vinegar and red pepper flakes.
5. Melt butter into the beef and vegetables.
6. Serve over brown rice and garnish with green onions.

8. Lemon-Balsamic Chicken Salad

Ingredients:

- 4 oz grilled chicken breast (chopped)
- ½ cup cooked quinoa
- 2 tablespoon extra virgin olive oil
- 1 cup mixed greens, diced cucumbers, and cherry tomatoes
- Garlic powder, thyme, and salt
- Balsamic vinegar
- Black pepper and parsley

Instructions:

1. Grill chicken and chop into bite-sized pieces.
2. Cook quinoa according to package instructions.
3. Arrange mixed greens, cucumbers, and cherry tomatoes in a bowl.
4. Add chicken and quinoa on top.
5. Drizzle with olive oil and balsamic vinegar.
6. Season with garlic powder, thyme, and salt.
7. Garnish with parsley and black pepper.

9. Chili-Lime Salmon and Brown Rice

Ingredients:

- 4 oz baked salmon
- ½ cup cooked brown rice
- 2 tablespoon grass-fed butter (melted)
- 1 cup roasted zucchini and asparagus
- Chili powder, lime zest, garlic powder, and salt
- Lime wedges

Instructions:

1. Season salmon with chili powder, lime zest, garlic powder, and salt.
2. Bake salmon until cooked through.

3. Cook brown rice according to package instructions.
4. Roast zucchini and asparagus until tender.
5. Drizzle melted butter over salmon.
6. Serve with brown rice, vegetables, and lime wedges.

10. Sardine Veggie Bowl with Quinoa

Ingredients:

- 1 can sardines (drained)
- ½ cup cooked quinoa
- 2 teaspoons extra virgin olive oil
- 1 cup roasted bell peppers, spinach, and red onions
- Paprika, garlic powder, and sea salt
- Lemon juice

Instructions:

1. Drain sardines and set aside.
2. Cook quinoa and mix with olive oil.
3. Roast bell peppers, spinach, and red onions until tender.
4. Season vegetables with paprika, garlic powder, and sea salt.
5. Combine quinoa and vegetables in a bowl.
6. Top with sardines and squeeze lemon juice before serving.

Recommended Resources

Limited Time Offer: FREE 30-minute Health Coach Consultation

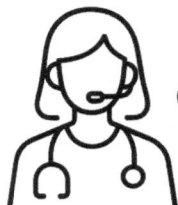

FREE
CONSULTATION
WITH
HEALTH COACH

GET STARTED

Check the Product's Ethics
cornucopia.org/scorecards

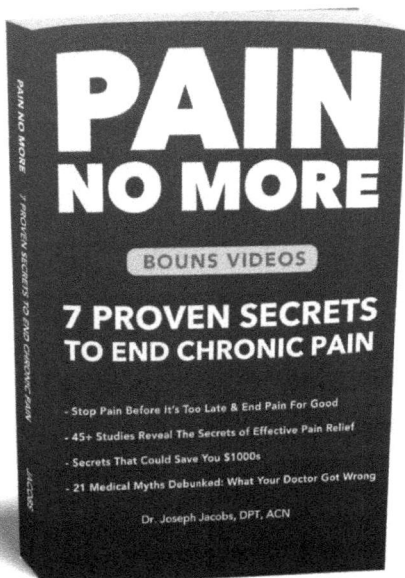

PAIN NO MORE

7 PROVEN SECRETS TO END CHRONIC PAIN

PAIN
NO MORE

BOUNS VIDEOS

7 PROVEN SECRETS
TO END CHRONIC PAIN

- Stop Pain Before It's Too Late & End Pain For Good
- 45+ Studies Reveal The Secrets of Effective Pain Relief
- Secrets That Could Save You $1000s
- 21 Medical Myths Debunked: What Your Doctor Got Wrong

Dr. Joseph Jacobs, DPT, ACN

BEATING
MIGRAINES

BONUS VIDEOS

7 NATURAL SECRETS FOR
LASTING RELIEF

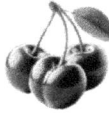

- End Migraines Naturally
- Clinically Proven Methods
- Treat the Root Cause, Not Symptoms
- Insights from a Doctor & Migraine Survivor
- Research-Backed Relief for Life

Dr. Joseph Jacobs, DPT, ACN

BEATING
ANXIETY
&
DEPRESSION

BONUS VIDEOS

14 NATURAL SECRETS TO
A HAPPIER LIFE

- Conquer Anxiety & Depression Naturally
- Heal the Root Causes & Reclaim Your Life
- Created by a Doctor Who Conquered PTSD & Depression
- Science-Based Strategies for Lasting Change

Dr. Joseph Jacobs, DPT, ACN

BEATING
BACK PAIN

BONUS VIDEOS

7 NATURAL SECRETS FOR
LASTING RELIEF

- End Back Pain Naturally
- Clinically Tested, Doctor-Approved
- Fix the Root Causes, Not Just Symptoms
- Backed by Science & Research
- Created by a Doctor Who Beat Chronic Pain

Dr. Joseph Jacobs, DPT, ACN

REVERSING
HIGH BLOOD
PRESSURE

7 NATURAL SECRETS TO SAFELY
LOWER BLOOD PRESSURE

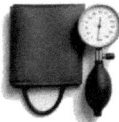

- Natural Solutions That Work
- Backed by Extensive Research
- Fix the Root Cause, Not Just the Numbers
- No Drugs, No Side Effects

Dr. Joseph Jacobs, DPT, ACN

181

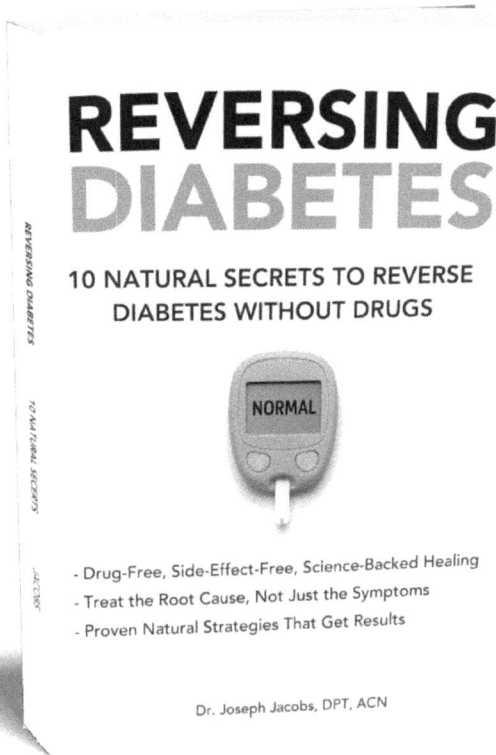

REVERSING DIABETES

10 NATURAL SECRETS TO REVERSE DIABETES WITHOUT DRUGS

NORMAL

- Drug-Free, Side-Effect-Free, Science-Backed Healing
- Treat the Root Cause, Not Just the Symptoms
- Proven Natural Strategies That Get Results

Dr. Joseph Jacobs, DPT, ACN

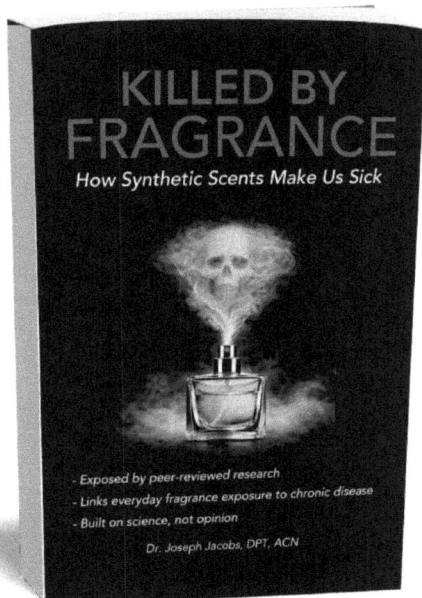

KILLED BY FRAGRANCE

How Synthetic Scents Make Us Sick

- Exposed by peer-reviewed research
- Links everyday fragrance exposure to chronic disease
- Built on science, not opinion

Dr. Joseph Jacobs, DPT, ACN

Your SHOES HURT YOU

Why Does Your Pain Keep Coming Back and *How to Fix It*

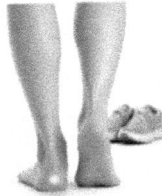

BONUS VIDEOS

- Fix Your Feet. Fix Your Pain.
- Why Modern Shoes Create Chronic Pain
- Backed by Biomechanics and Clinical Research

Dr. Joseph Jacobs, DPT, ACN

Glossary

Antibiotic Resistance: A reduced response to antibiotic medications caused by overuse or misuse, allowing bacteria to survive and become harder to treat.

Antioxidants: Protective compounds found in foods such as fruits, vegetables, nuts, and seeds that help neutralize free radicals and reduce oxidative stress.

Atkins Diet: A low-carbohydrate diet that progresses through phases, beginning with strict carbohydrate restriction and gradually increasing carbohydrate intake over time.

Autoimmune Disorders: Conditions in which the immune system mistakenly attacks the body's own tissues, often influenced by chronic inflammation, genetics, and environmental triggers.

Bioavailable Nutrients: Nutrients the body can absorb and use efficiently, most commonly found in whole, minimally processed foods.

BMI (Body Mass Index): A screening measurement based on height and weight used to estimate body weight status, including underweight, normal weight, overweight, or obesity.

Calcium Deficiency: Inadequate calcium intake, which can weaken bones and increase the risk of fractures and osteoporosis.

Cardiovascular Diseases: Disorders of the heart and blood vessels, including coronary artery disease, heart attack, and stroke.

Carnivore Diet: A highly restrictive eating pattern that eliminates plant foods and consists only of animal-based foods such as meat, fish, eggs, and animal fats.

Chlorination Byproducts: Chemicals formed when chlorine used in water treatment reacts with organic materials, including compounds such as trihalomethanes.

Chronic Disease Prevention: Lifestyle strategies that reduce long-term disease risk, including nutrition, physical activity, sleep, and stress regulation.

Chronic Inflammation: A prolonged inflammatory response that can damage tissues and contribute to diabetes, heart disease, autoimmune dysfunction, and other chronic conditions.

Collagen: A structural protein that supports skin, joints, tendons, ligaments, bones, and connective tissue strength.

DASH Diet: A dietary pattern originally designed to reduce high blood pressure, emphasizing fruits, vegetables, whole grains, lean proteins, and low-fat dairy while limiting sodium and processed foods.

Detox Diet: A dietary program that claims to remove toxins from the body, often involving calorie restriction, supplements, or elimination of multiple food groups.

Dietary Fiber: A plant-based carbohydrate that supports digestion, gut health, cholesterol balance, and blood sugar regulation.

Disinfection Byproducts (DBPs): Chemicals formed when disinfectants such as chlorine or chloramine react with organic matter in water.

Electrolytes: Minerals such as sodium, potassium, and magnesium that support hydration, nerve signaling, and muscle function.

Endocrine Disruptors: Chemicals found in some plastics, pesticides, and consumer products that may interfere with hormone signaling in the body.

Fasting Window: The period of time during intermittent fasting when no calories are consumed.

Flavonoids: Plant compounds with antioxidant and anti-inflammatory effects found in foods such as berries, citrus, tea, and leafy greens.

Fruitarian Diet: An extreme plant-based eating pattern focused primarily on fruit, often excluding most other foods such as grains, legumes, and protein-rich sources.

Glucose Intolerance: A reduced ability to process blood sugar effectively, often considered an early stage of insulin resistance.

Gut Microbiota: The community of microorganisms living in the digestive tract that supports digestion, immune function, and inflammation regulation.

Heart Disease: A broad term for conditions affecting heart structure or function, including coronary artery disease and heart failure.

Healthy Fats: Fats that support cellular and cardiovascular health, including monounsaturated and polyunsaturated fats.

Heavy Metals: Toxic elements such as lead, mercury, cadmium, and arsenic that can contaminate food or water and harm the nervous system and organs.

Hydration: Maintaining adequate body fluid levels to support digestion, metabolism, temperature regulation, circulation, and cellular function.

Inflammation: The body's protective immune response to injury or infection that becomes harmful when excessive or chronic.

Intermittent Fasting (IF): An eating pattern that alternates between scheduled eating periods and fasting periods.

Juice Cleanse: A restrictive diet that replaces meals with fruit and vegetable juices for a set period, often lacking adequate protein and fiber.

Ketogenic Diet: A very low-carbohydrate, high-fat diet designed to shift the body into ketosis, where fat-derived ketones become a primary fuel source.

Macronutrients: The three major nutrients needed in large amounts for energy and body function: carbohydrates, proteins, and fats.

Mediterranean Diet: A dietary pattern emphasizing vegetables, fruits, legumes, whole grains, olive oil, and fish, commonly associated with heart-health benefits.

Mental Health Disorders: Conditions affecting mood, thinking, or behavior, including anxiety, depression, and related disorders.

Micronutrients: Vitamins and minerals needed in small amounts to support immunity, metabolism, bone health, and energy production.

Microplastics: Tiny plastic particles found in food, water, and the environment that may accumulate in the body.

Glossary

Non-GMO Foods: Foods produced without genetic modification, often chosen for cleaner sourcing and fewer agricultural chemical exposures.

Nutrient Deficiency: Inadequate intake or absorption of essential nutrients, which can contribute to fatigue, weakened immunity, and impaired organ function.

Nutrient-Dense Foods: Foods rich in vitamins, minerals, and protective compounds relative to their calorie content.

Obesity: A medical condition characterized by excess body fat, commonly defined as a BMI of 30 or higher.

Omega-3 Fatty Acids: Essential fats that support brain, heart, and inflammatory balance, found in fatty fish, flax, chia, and walnuts.

Overweight: A weight classification commonly defined by a BMI between 25.0 and 29.9.

Paleo Diet: An eating pattern based on whole foods such as meats, fish, vegetables, fruits, nuts, and seeds while excluding grains, legumes, and most dairy.

Phytonutrients: Naturally occurring plant compounds that support antioxidant activity, inflammation regulation, and immune defense.

Pesticides: Agricultural chemicals used to control pests, which may remain as residues on food and contribute to health risks with chronic exposure.

Polychlorinated Biphenyls (PCBs): Persistent industrial pollutants that can accumulate in animal tissue, including certain fish, and may affect immune and endocrine function.

Processed Foods: Foods altered from their natural form through manufacturing, such as refining, preservatives, additives, or industrial preparation.

Probiotics: Live beneficial microorganisms that support digestive health and microbiome balance.

Pro-inflammatory Foods: Foods associated with increased inflammation, including refined sugars, processed meats, trans fats, and ultra-processed foods.

Raw Vegan Diet: A plant-based diet consisting primarily of uncooked foods, often excluding cooked vegetables, grains, legumes, and all animal products.

Refined Carbohydrates: Carbohydrates stripped of fiber and nutrients during processing, such as white bread and sugary snacks, which can spike blood sugar.

Saturated Fats: A type of fat found in animal foods and certain oils that may raise LDL cholesterol when consumed excessively.

Seed Oils: Highly processed oils made from seeds such as soybean, sunflower, and canola, often high in omega-6 fats.

Systemic Inflammation: Low-grade inflammation throughout the body that may contribute to chronic disease development.

Thermal Processing: Heat-based food processing methods such as pasteurization that can reduce certain heat-sensitive nutrients.

Glossary

Toxin-Free Diet: A nutrition approach that minimizes chemical exposures and additives by prioritizing clean, whole foods.

Type 2 Diabetes: A chronic metabolic condition characterized by insulin resistance and elevated blood sugar levels.

Ultra-Processed Foods (UPFs): Industrial foods made with refined ingredients and additives that are associated with metabolic dysfunction and chronic disease risk.

Vegan Diet: A plant-based eating pattern that eliminates all animal-derived foods, including meat, dairy, eggs, and fish.

Vitamin D Deficiency: Low vitamin D levels that may affect bone strength, immune function, and overall health.

Whole30 Diet: A 30-day elimination diet that removes added sugars, alcohol, grains, dairy, legumes, and additives, followed by structured reintroduction.

References

1. Centers for Disease Control and Prevention (CDC). Overweight and Obesity Statistics. Updated May 17, 2022. https://www.cdc.gov/nchs/fastats/obesity-overweight.htm

2. Centers for Disease Control and Prevention (CDC). Adult Obesity Facts. Updated October 7, 2022. https://www.cdc.gov/obesity/adult-obesity-facts/index.html

3. Centers for Disease Control and Prevention (CDC). Youth Obesity Trends: Prevalence and Disparities. Updated October 13, 2023. https://www.cdc.gov/mmwr/volumes/73/wr/mm7341a5.htm

4. New York Post. Obesity Rates in the US Not Growing for First Time in a Decade, But Severe Obesity is Rising: CDC. Published September 24, 2024. https://nypost.com/2024/09/24/lifestyle/obesity-rates-in-us-not-growing-for-first-time-in-a-decade-but-severe-obesity-on-the-rise-cdc/

5. New York Post. America is Fatter Than Ever: These States Tip the Scales on Obesity. Published September 13, 2024. https://nypost.com/2024/09/13/lifestyle/america-is-fatter-than-ever-these-states-tip-the-scales-on-obesity/

6. Saltiel AR, Olefsky JM. Inflammatory mechanisms linking obesity and metabolic disease. *J Clin Invest*. 2017;127(1):1-4. doi:10.1172/JCI92035.

7. Ng M, Fleming T, Robinson M, et al. Global, regional, and national prevalence of overweight and obesity in children and adults during 1980–2013: a systematic analysis for the Global Burden of Disease Study 2013. *Lancet*.2014;384(9945):766-781. doi:10.1016/S0140-6736(14)60460-8.

8. Farrell GC, Wong VW, Chitturi S. NAFLD in Asia—as common and important as in the West. *Nat Rev Gastroenterol Hepatol*. 2013;10(5):307-318. doi:10.1038/nrgastro.2013.34.

9. Després JP, Lemieux I. Abdominal obesity and metabolic syndrome. *Nature*. 2006;444(7121):881-887. doi:10.1038/nature05488.

10. Grundy SM. Metabolic syndrome pandemic. *Arterioscler Thromb Vasc Biol*. 2008;28(4):629-636. doi:10.1161/ATVBAHA.107.151092.

11. Pereira-Santos M, Costa PR, Assis AM, Santos CA, Santos DB. Obesity and vitamin D deficiency: A systematic review and meta-analysis. *Obes Rev*. 2015;16(4):341-349. doi:10.1111/obr.12239.

12. Cepeda-Lopez AC, Osendarp SJ, Melse-Boonstra A, et al. Sharpening the double-edged sword: A systematic review and meta-analysis of the evidence for a causal relationship between iron deficiency and obesity. *Obes Rev*.2015;16(8):751-762. doi:10.1111/obr.12299.

13. Barbagallo M, Dominguez LJ. Magnesium and type 2 diabetes. *World J Diabetes*. 2015;6(10):1152-1157. doi:10.4239/wjd.v6.i10.1152.

14. Al-Marzooqi W, Abotalib Z, Zaidi S. Zinc and obesity: Molecular and biochemical evidence. *World J Metab Syndr*.2019;8(3):18-27. doi:10.5414/IBP.2015.0058.

15. Devalia V. Folate and vitamin B12 deficiency: An overview of the mechanisms of anemia in the elderly. *Nutrition*.2006;22(5):447-455. doi:10.1016/j.nut.2005.10.015.

16. Zemel MB. Role of calcium and dairy products in energy partitioning and weight management. *Am J Clin Nutr*.2004;79(5):907S-912S. doi:10.1093/ajcn/79.5.907S.

17. Rafiq S, Jeppesen PB. Is hypovitaminosis D a consequence of obesity? *Clin Endocrinol (Oxf)*. 2018;89(1):35-48. doi:10.1111/cen.13724.

References

18. Cepeda-Lopez AC, Osendarp SJ, Melse-Boonstra A, et al. Iron bioavailability is reduced in overweight and obese women. *Am J Clin Nutr.* 2011;93(5):1092-1101. doi:10.3945/ajcn.110.007195.

19. Drewnowski A, Almiron-Roig E. Human perceptions and preferences for fat-rich foods. *Obes Rev.* 2010;11(6):454-467. doi:10.1111/j.1467-789X.2010.00717.x.

20. World Health Organization (WHO). Malnutrition. Published June 9, 2021. https://www.who.int/news-room/fact-sheets/detail/malnutrition

21. Gearhardt AN, Davis C, Kuschner R, Brownell KD. The addiction potential of hyperpalatable foods. *Curr Drug Abuse Rev.* 2011;4(3):140-145. doi:10.2174/1874473711104030140

22. Adam TC, Epel ES. Stress, eating and the reward system. *Physiol Behav.* 2007;91(4):449-458. doi:10.1016/j.physbeh.2007.04.011

23. Volkow ND, Wang GJ, Fowler JS, Telang F. Overlapping neuronal circuits in addiction and obesity: evidence of systems pathology. *Philos Trans R Soc Lond B Biol Sci.* 2008;363(1507):3191-3200. doi:10.1098/rstb.2008.0107

24. Hebebrand J, Albayrak Ö, Adan R, et al. "Eating addiction", rather than "food addiction", better captures addictive-like eating behavior. *Neurosci Biobehav Rev.* 2014;47:295-306. doi:10.1016/j.neubiorev.2014.08.016

25. Yannakoulia M, Panagiotakos DB, Pitsavos C, et al. Eating habits in relations to anxiety symptoms among apparently healthy adults: A pattern analysis from the ATTICA Study. *Appetite.* 2008;51(3):519-525. doi:10.1016/j.appet.2008.04.002

26. Lustig RH. Fructose: metabolic, hedonic, and societal parallels with ethanol. *J Am Diet Assoc.* 2010;110(9):1307-1321. doi:10.1016/j.jada.2010.06.008

27. Puhl RM, Latner JD. Stigma, obesity, and the health of the nation's children. *Psychol Bull.* 2007;133(4):557-580. doi:10.1037/0033-2909.133.4.557

28. Selye H. Stress and the general adaptation syndrome. *Br Med J.* 1950;1(4667):1383-1392. doi:10.1136/bmj.1.4667.1383

29. Volkow ND, Wang GJ, Tomasi D, Baler RD. Obesity and addiction: Neurobiological overlaps. *Obes Rev.*2013;14(1):2-18. doi:10.1111/j.1467-789X.2012.01031.x.\

30. Stice E, Spoor S, Bohon C, Small DM. Relation between obesity and blunted striatal response to food is moderated by TaqlA A1 allele. *Science.* 2008;322(5900):449-452. doi:10.1126/science.1161550.

31. Kenny PJ. Reward mechanisms in obesity: New insights and future directions. *Neuron.* 2011;69(4):664-679. doi:10.1016/j.neuron.2011.02.016.

32. Klok MD, Jakobsdottir S, Drent ML. The role of leptin and ghrelin in the regulation of food intake and body weight in humans: A review. *Obes Rev.* 2007;8(1):21-34. doi:10.1111/j.1467-789X.2006.00270.x.

33. Müller TD, Nogueiras R, Andermann ML, et al. Ghrelin. *Mol Metab.* 2015;4(6):437-460. doi:10.1016/j.molmet.2015.03.005.

34. Farr OM, Tsoukas MA, Mantzoros CS. Leptin and the brain: Influences on brain development, cognitive functioning and psychiatric disorders. *Metabolism.* 2015;64(1):114-130. doi:10.1016/j.metabol.2014.10.013.

35. Davis C, Levitan RD, Kaplan AS, et al. Dopamine for "wanting" and opioids for "liking": A comparison of obese adults with and without binge eating. *Obesity (Silver Spring).* 2009;17(6):1220-1225. doi:10.1038/oby.2009.52.

References

36. Cornelis MC, Rimm EB, Curhan GC, Kraft P, Hunter DJ, Hu FB. Obesity susceptibility loci and uncontrolled eating, emotional eating and cognitive restraint behaviors in men and women. *Obesity (Silver Spring)*.2014;22(5):E135-E141. doi:10.1002/oby.20723.

37. Stoeckel LE, Weller RE, Cook EW, Twieg DB, Knowlton RC, Cox JE. Widespread reward-system activation in obese women in response to pictures of high-calorie foods. *NeuroImage*. 2008;41(2):636-647. doi:10.1016/j.neuroimage.2008.02.031.

38. Gearhardt AN, Corbin WR, Brownell KD. Food addiction: An examination of the diagnostic criteria for dependence. *J Addict Med*. 2009;3(1):1-7. doi:10.1097/ADM.0b013e318193c993.

39. Volkow ND, Wise RA. How can drug addiction help us understand obesity? *Nat Neurosci*. 2005;8(5):555-560. doi:10.1038/nn1452.

40. Mason AE, Jhaveri K, Cohn M, et al. Reduced reward-driven eating accounts for the impact of a mindfulness-based diet and exercise intervention on weight loss: Data from the SHINE randomized controlled trial. *Appetite*. 2016;100:86-93. doi:10.1016/j.appet.2016.02.009.

41. Berthoud HR. Interactions between the "cognitive" and "metabolic" brain in the control of food intake. *Physiol Behav*.2007;91(5):486-498. doi:10.1016/j.physbeh.2006.12.016.

42. Inoue S, Zimmet P, Caterson I, et al. The Asia-Pacific perspective: Redefining obesity and its treatment. *Health Communications Australia Pty Limited*. 2000.

43. Adam TC, Epel ES. Stress, eating and the reward system. *Physiol Behav*. 2007;91(4):449-458. doi:10.1016/j.physbeh.2007.04.011.

44. Apolzan JW, Bray GA, Smith SR, et al. Effects of weight gain induced by controlled overfeeding on physical activity. *Am J Physiol Endocrinol Metab*. 2014;307(11):E1030-E1037. doi:10.1152/ajpendo.00239.2014.

45. Gearhardt AN, Boswell RG, White MA. The association of "food addiction" with disordered eating and body mass index. *Eat Behav*. 2014;15(3):427-433. doi:10.1016/j.eatbeh.2014.04.001.'

46. Adam TC, Epel ES. Stress, eating and the reward system. *Physiol Behav*. 2007;91(4):449-458. doi:10.1016/j.physbeh.2007.04.011.

47. Finlayson G, King N, Blundell JE. Liking vs. wanting food: Importance for human appetite control and weight regulation. *Neurosci Biobehav Rev*. 2007;31(3):987-1002. doi:10.1016/j.neubiorev.2007.03.004.

48. Pecoraro N, Reyes TM, Gomez F, Bhargava A, Dallman MF. Chronic stress promotes palatable feeding, which reduces signs of stress: Feedforward and feedback effects of chronic stress. *Endocrinology*. 2004;145(8):3754-3762. doi:10.1210/en.2004-0305.

49. van Strien T, Herman CP, Anschutz DJ, Engels RC, de Weerth C. Moderation of distress-induced eating by emotional eating scores. *Appetite*. 2012;58(1):277-284. doi:10.1016/j.appet.2011.10.005.

50. Karlsson J, Persson LO, Sjöström L, Sullivan M. Psychometric properties and factor structure of the Three-Factor Eating Questionnaire (TFEQ) in obese men and women. *Results from the Swedish Obese Subjects (SOS) study*. Int J Obes Relat Metab Disord. 2000;24(12):1715-1725. doi:10.1038/sj.ijo.0801442.

References

51. Hebebrand J, Albayrak O, Adan R, et al. "Eating addiction," rather than "food addiction," better captures addictive-like eating behavior. *Neurosci Biobehav Rev.* 2014;47:295-306. doi:10.1016/j.neubiorev.2014.08.016.

52. U.S. Food and Drug Administration (FDA). Overview of Food Ingredients, Additives & Colors. Updated November 15, 2022. https://www.fda.gov/food/food-additives-petitions/overview-food-ingredients-additives-colors

53. European Food Safety Authority (EFSA). Food Additives. Published 2022. https://www.efsa.europa.eu/en/topics/topic/food-additives

54. European Commission. The EU Precautionary Principle: Ensuring Safety in the Face of Scientific Uncertainty.

55. Codex Alimentarius Commission. General Standard for Food Additives. Joint FAO/WHO Food Standards Program. https://www.fao.org/fao-who-codexalimentarius

56. Davis DR, Epp MD, Riordan HD. Changes in USDA Food Composition Data for 43 Garden Crops, 1950 to 1999. *J Am Coll Nutr.* 2004;23(6):669-682. doi:10.1080/07315724.2004.10719409.

57. Mayer AM. Historical Changes in the Mineral Content of Fruits and Vegetables. *Br Food J.* 1997;99(6):207-211. doi:10.1108/00070709710181540.

58. White PJ, Broadley MR. Historical Variation in the Mineral Composition of Edible Horticultural Products. *J Hortic Sci Biotechnol.* 2005;80(6):660-667. doi:10.1080/14620316.2005.1151197

59. Fan MS, Zhao FJ, Fairweather-Tait SJ, Poulton PR, McGrath SP. Evidence of Decreasing Mineral Density in Wheat Grain Over the Last 160 Years. *J Trace Elem Med Biol.* 2008;22(4):315-324. doi:10.1016/j.jtemb.2008.07.002

60. The Food Untold. How Nutrient Loss Occurs in Fruits and Vegetables. Published 2007. https://thefooduntold.com/health/how-nutrient-loss-occurs-in-fruits-and-vegetables/

61. Livestrong. How Do Fruits and Vegetables Lose Their Nutrients After Picking? Published 2021. https://www.livestrong.com/article/447449-how-do-fruits-and-vegetables-lose-their-nutrients-after-picking/

62. Journals of the American Society for Horticultural Science. Historical Declines in Mineral Nutrients in Produce. Published 2005.https://journals.ashs.org/hortsci/view/journals/hortsci/44/1/article-p15.xml

63. University of California Agriculture and Natural Resources. Postharvest Handling and Storage Practices to Minimize Nutrient Loss. Published 2016.

64. Owens FN, Secrist DS, Hill WJ, Gill DR. Acidosis in cattle: A review. *J Anim Sci.* 1998;76(1):275-286. doi:10.2527/1998.761275x

65. Nagaraja TG, Lechtenberg KF. Liver abscesses in feedlot cattle. *Vet Clin Food Anim.* 2007;23(2):351-369. doi:10.1016/j.cvfa.2007.05.002

66. Krause KM, Oetzel GR. Understanding and preventing subacute ruminal acidosis in dairy herds: A review. *J Dairy Sci.* 2006;89(4):139-159. doi:10.3168/jds.S0022-0302(06)72194-0

67. Brown EG, et al. The effects of grain-based diets on cattle health. *Front Vet Sci.* 2018;5:245. doi:10.3389/fvets.2018.00245

68. Henderson DC, et al. Nutritional implications of grain-fed diets in livestock. *Anim Reprod Sci.* 2021;230:106834. doi:10.1016/j.anireprosci.2021.106834

References

69. Nourish Cooperative. Grass-Fed vs. Grain-Fed Beef: Why Grass-Fed is better for your health. Published November 2, 2024.. https://nourishcooperative.com/blog/grass-fed-vs-grain-fed-beef-why-grass-fed-is-better-for-your-health

70. Global Research. The True Impact of Grass Fed Beef: Why Your Meat's Origin Matters More Than Ever. Published December 2024. https://www.globalresearch.ca/true-impact-grass-fed-beef/5873122

71. The Organic Center. The environmental and health impacts of growth hormones in cattle rearing. Published December 2013. https://www.organic-center.org/research/environmental-and-health-impacts-growth-hormones-cattle-rearing

72. Heart & Soil. Grass-Fed vs Grain-Fed Beef: Which is Best? Published July 2023. 2025. https://heartandsoil.co/blog/grass-fed-vs-grain-fed-beef/

73. Cleveland Clinic. Cleveland Clinic study finds common artificial sweetener linked to higher rates of heart attack and stroke. Published February 27, 2023. https://newsroom.clevelandclinic.org/2023/02/27/cleveland-clinic-study-finds-common-artificial-sweetener-linked-to-higher-rates-of-heart-attack-and-stroke

74. Debras C, Chazelas E, Srour B, et al. Artificial sweeteners and risk of cardiovascular diseases: results from the NutriNet-Santé cohort. *BMJ*. 2022;378:e071204. doi:10.1136/bmj-2022-071204

75. Touvier M, Chazelas E, Deschasaux M, et al. Consumption of artificial sweeteners and cancer risk: Results from the NutriNet-Santé cohort. *PLoS Med*. 2022;19(8):e1003950. doi:10.1371/journal.pmed.1003950

76. Harvard Health Publishing. Could artificial sweeteners be bad for your brain? Published June 7, 2017. https://www.health.harvard.edu/blog/could-artificial-sweeteners-be-bad-for-your-brain-2017060711849

77. Suez J, Korem T, Zeevi D, et al. Artificial sweeteners induce glucose intolerance by altering the gut microbiota. *Nature*. 2014;514(7521):181-186. doi:10.1038/nature13793

78. Food & Wine. This Popular Artificial Sweetener Is Linked to Heart Attacks and Strokes, Research Shows. Published February 2023. https://www.foodandwine.com/erythritol-heart-attack-stroke-study-8694329

79. Crimson Publishers. Nutritional Losses During Food Processing: A Review. Published 2023. https://crimsonpublishers.com/mcda/fulltext/MCDA.000783.php

80. Cambridge University Press. Nutritional Losses and Gains During Processing: Future Problems and Issues. *Proceedings of the Nutrition Society*. Published 2023. https://www.cambridge.org/core/journals/proceedings-of-the-nutrition-society/article/nutritional-losses-and-gains-during-processing-future-problems-and-issues/736B380C57416E2B8185272158AE8E71

81. Verywell Health. Are Fresh or Frozen Vegetables More Nutritious? Published November 2023. https://www.verywellhealth.com/frozen-vs-fresh-vegetables-8663723

82. Sanders ME, Merenstein DJ, Reid G, Gibson GR, Rastall RA. Probiotics and Prebiotics in Intestinal Health and Disease: From Biology to the Clinic. *Nat Rev Gastroenterol Hepatol*. 2019;16(10):605-616. doi:10.1038/s41575-019-0173-3.

83. Sah B, Vasiljevic T, McKechnie S, Donkor ON. Effect of Bacterial Interactions on the Viability of Probiotic Bacteria in Dairy Products Under Heat Treatment and Refrigerated Storage. *J Food Sci*. 2015;80(12):M3023-M3030. doi:10.1111/1750-3841.13156.

References

84. Gueimonde M, Ouwehand AC, Salminen S. Safety of Probiotic Bacteria. *Asia Pac J Clin Nutr.* 2006;15(4):551-558. doi:10.1108/00070700810877964.

85. Champagne CP, Ross RP, Saarela M, Hansen KF, Charalampopoulos D. Recommendations for the Viability Assessment of Probiotics as Concentrated Cultures and in Food Matrices. *Int J Food Microbiol.* 2011;149(3):185-193. doi:10.1016/j.ijfoodmicro.2011.07.005.

86. Anandharaj M, Sivasankari B. Isolation of Potential Probiotic Lactobacillus Strains from Human Milk. *Int J Res Stud Biosci.* 2014;2(4):19-27. https://www.arcjournals.org/pdfs/ijrsb/v2-i4/4.pdf

87. Harvard T.H. Chan School of Public Health. Shining the Spotlight on Trans Fats. https://nutritionsource.hsph.harvard.edu/what-should-you-eat/fats-and-cholesterol/types-of-fat/transfats/

88. World Health Organization. Nutrition: Trans Fat. https://www.who.int/news-room/questions-and-answers/item/nutrition-trans-fat

89. American Heart Association. Trans Fats. https://www.heart.org/en/healthy-living/healthy-eating/eat-smart/fats/trans-fat

90. The BMJ. Intake of Saturated and Trans Unsaturated Fatty Acids and Risk of All-Cause Mortality. https://www.bmj.com/content/351/bmj.h3978

91. Centers for Disease Control and Prevention. Global Surveillance of Trans-Fatty Acids. https://www.cdc.gov/pcd/issues/2019/19_0121.htm

92. The American Journal of Clinical Nutrition. Health Effects of Trans Fatty Acids. https://ajcn.nutrition.org/article/S0002-9165%2823%2918043-9/fulltext

93. European Heart Journal. Natural Trans Fat, Dairy Fat, Partially Hydrogenated Oils, and Cardiovascular Health. https://academic.oup.com/eurheartj/article/37/13/1079/2398446

94. WebMD. Trans Fats: The Science and the Risks. https://www.webmd.com/diet/features/trans-fats-science-and-risks

95. Wikipedia. Trans Fat. https://en.wikipedia.org/wiki/Trans_fat

96. Wikipedia. Fat Hydrogenation. https://en.wikipedia.org/wiki/Fat_hydrogenation

97. Thomas D. A Study on the Mineral Depletion of the Foods Available to Us as a Nation Over the Period 1940 to 2002. *Nutr Health.* 2007;19(1-2):21-55. doi:10.1177/026010600701900205.

98. Jarrell WM, Beverly RL. The Dilution Effect in Plant Nutrition Studies. *Adv Agron.* 1981;34:197-224. doi:10.1016/S0065-2113(08)60887-1.

99. World Health Organization (WHO). Endocrine Disruptors and Human Health. Published 2023. https://www.who.int/news-room/fact-sheets/detail/endocrine-disruptors

100. U.S. Food and Drug Administration (FDA). Bisphenol A (BPA): Use in Food Contact Applications. Updated January 2025. https://www.fda.gov/food/food-additives-petitions/bisphenol-bpa-information

101. Centers for Disease Control and Prevention (CDC). Per- and Polyfluoroalkyl Substances (PFAS) Factsheet. Updated December 2024. https://www.cdc.gov/chemical/pfas/index.html

102. European Food Safety Authority (EFSA). Risks for Human Health Related to the Presence of Mineral Oil Hydrocarbons in Food. Published 2022. https://www.efsa.europa.eu/en/news/risk-assessment-mineral-oil-hydrocarbons-food

References

103. International Agency for Research on Cancer (IARC). Formaldehyde Classification as a Carcinogen. Updated 2022. https://monographs.iarc.who.int/agents/formaldehyde/

104. U.S. Environmental Protection Agency (EPA). Phthalates Action Plan. Published 2021. https://www.epa.gov/assessing-and-managing-chemicals-under-tsca/phthalates

105. Monteiro CA, Cannon G, Levy RB, et al. Ultra-processed Foods: What They Are and How to Identify Them. *Public Health Nutr.* 2019;22(5):936-941. doi:10.1017/S1368980018003762.

106. Fiolet T, Srour B, Sellem L, et al. Consumption of Ultra-processed Foods and Cancer Risk: Results From NutriNet-Santé Prospective Cohort. *BMJ.* 2018;360:k322. doi:10.1136/bmj.k322.

107. World Health Organization (WHO). Healthy Diet: The Dangers of Ultra-Processed Foods. Updated 2023. https://www.who.int/news-room/fact-sheets/detail/healthy-diet

108. Harvard T.H. Chan School of Public Health. Processed Foods and Health: The Risks of Overconsumption. Published 2024. https://www.hsph.harvard.edu/nutritionsource/processed-foods

109. Mayo Clinic. Ultra-Processed Foods and Health Risks: Understanding Their Impact. Published 2022. https://www.mayoclinic.org/processed-foods

110. National Institute of Diabetes and Digestive and Kidney Diseases (NIDDK). Definition and Facts for Lactose Intolerance. Updated March 2023. https://www.niddk.nih.gov/health-information/digestive-diseases/lactose-intolerance/definition-facts

111. Wikipedia. Lactose Intolerance. Updated December 2024. https://en.wikipedia.org/wiki/Lactose_intolerance

112. Storhaug CL, Fosse SK, Fadnes LT. Country, Regional, and Global Estimates for Lactose Malabsorption in Adults: A Systematic Review and Meta-Analysis. *Lancet Gastroenterol Hepatol.* 2017;2(10):738-746. doi:10.1016/S2468-1253(17)30154-1.

113. Patterson RE, Sears DD. Metabolic Effects of Intermittent Fasting. *Annu Rev Nutr.* 2017;37:371-393. doi:10.1146/annurev-nutr-071816-064634.

114. Harvie M, Howell A. Potential Benefits and Harms of Intermittent Energy Restriction and Intermittent Fasting Diets. *Obes Res Clin Pract.* 2017;11(1):90-99. doi:10.1016/j.orcp.2016.08.002.

115. Mattson MP, Longo VD, Harvie M. Impact of Intermittent Fasting on Health and Disease Processes. *Ageing Res Rev.* 2017;39:46-58. doi:10.1016/j.arr.2016.10.005.

116. de Cabo R, Mattson MP. Effects of Intermittent Fasting on Health, Aging, and Disease. *N Engl J Med.* 2019;381(26):2541-2551. doi:10.1056/NEJMra1905136.

117. Tinsley GM, La Bounty PM. Effects of Intermittent Fasting on Body Composition and Clinical Health Markers in Humans. *Nutr Rev.* 2015;73(10):661-674. doi:10.1093/nutrit/nuv041.

118. Manoogian EN, Panda S. Circadian rhythms, time-restricted feeding, and healthy aging. *Ageing Res Rev.*;39:59-67. doi:10.1016/j.arr.2016.12.006.

119. National Academies of Sciences, Engineering, and Medicine. Dietary Reference Intakes for Water, Potassium, Sodium, Chloride, and Sulfate. National Academies Press; 2005. doi:10.17226/10925.

120. Popkin BM, D'Anci KE, Rosenberg IH. Water, Hydration, and Health. *Nutr Rev.* 2010;68(8):439-458. doi:10.1111/j.1753-4887.2010.00304.x.

References

121. Centers for Disease Control and Prevention (CDC). Get the Facts: Drinking Water and Your Health. Updated June 6, 2022. https://www.cdc.gov/healthywater/drinking/nutrition/index.html
122. Mayo Clinic. Water: How Much Should You Drink Every Day? Published 2023. https://www.mayoclinic.org/healthy-lifestyle/nutrition-and-healthy-eating/expert-answers/water/faq-20058345
123. Armstrong LE, Johnson EC. Water Intake, Water Balance, and the Elusive Daily Water Requirement. *Nutrients*. 2018;10(12):1928. doi:10.3390/nu10121928.
124. U.S. Geological Survey. Tap water study detects PFAS 'forever chemicals' across the US. Published July 5, 2023.
125. Quinete N, Hauser-Davis RA. Drinking water pollutants may affect the immune system: concerns regarding COVID-19 health effects. *Environ Sci Pollut Res Int*. 2020;27(30):37519-37530.
126. Harvard T.H. Chan School of Public Health. Communities of color disproportionately exposed to PFAS pollution in drinking water. Published May 15, 2023.
127. U.S. Geological Survey. Tap water study detects PFAS "forever chemicals" across the US. Published July 5, 2023. https://www.usgs.gov/news/national-news-release/tap-water-study-detects-pfas-forever-chemicals-across-us
128. Le Monde. Drinking water in Paris and other European cities contaminated with an unmonitored 'forever chemical'. Published July 10, 2024. https://www.lemonde.fr/en/environment/article/2024/07/10/drinking-water-in-paris-and-other-european-cities-contaminated-with-an-unmonitored-forever-chemical_6679968_114.html
129. Post T. 'Mystery' chemical found in millions of Americans' tap water could be toxic: 'Good reason to investigate'. Published November 22, 2024. https://nypost.com/2024/11/22/lifestyle/mystery-chemical-found-in-american-tap-water-may-be-toxic
130. PLOS ONE. Microplastic contamination in tap water, beer, and sea salt. Published March 23, 2018. https://journals.plos.org/plosone/article?id=10.1371%2Fjournal.pone.0194970
131. Yahoo News. Study raises more questions about fluoride levels and cognitive effects. Published October 10, 2024. https://www.yahoo.com/news/study-raises-more-questions-fluoride-003449791.html
132. United States Environmental Protection Agency. *Water Treatment Systems: Types and Effectiveness*. Published 2023.
133. World Health Organization. Guidelines for Drinking-water Quality. 4th ed. Geneva: WHO; 2022.
134. Shrestha A, Smith WA. Performance of household water treatment systems: A critical review. *J Water Health*. 2020;18(3):317-328.
135. National Sanitation Foundation (NSF). *Standards and Testing for Water Filters*.
136. National Center for Complementary and Integrative Health (NCCIH). Herbs at a Glance. Updated December 2024. https://www.nccih.nih.gov/health/herbsataglance
137. McKay DL, Blumberg JB. A Review of the Bioactivity and Potential Health Benefits of Chamomile Tea (Matricaria recutita L.). *Phytother Res*. 2006;20(7):519-530. doi:10.1002/ptr.1900.

References

138. Heck CI, de Mejia EG. Yerba Mate Tea (Ilex paraguariensis): A Comprehensive Review on Chemistry, Health Implications, and Technological Considerations. *J Food Sci.* 2007;72(9):R138-R151. doi:10.1111/j.1750-3841.2007.00535.x.

139. Singh R, Sharma P, Malviya R. Echinacea: A Source of Bioactive Constituents and a Popular Herbal Remedy. *Pharmacogn Rev.* 2012;6(11):95-103. doi:10.4103/0973-7847.95883.

140. Ng QX, Venkatanarayanan N, Ho CY. Clinical Use of Lemon Balm (Melissa officinalis) for Anxiety and Other Neuropsychiatric Conditions. *Phytother Res.* 2018;32(3):437-445. doi:10.1002/ptr.5997.

141. Akilen R, Tsiami A, Devendra D, Robinson N. Glycated Haemoglobin and Blood Pressure-Lowering Effect of Cinnamon in Multi-Ethnic Type 2 Diabetic Patients in the UK: A Randomised, Placebo-Controlled, Double-Blind Clinical Trial. *Diabet Med.* 2010;27(10):1159-1167. doi:10.1111/j.1464-5491.2010.03079.x.

142. Kennedy DO, Scholey AB. The Psychopharmacology of European Herbs with Cognition-Enhancing Properties. *Curr Pharm Des.* 2006;12(35):4613-4623. doi:10.2174/138161206778887032.

143. Gardner EJ, Ruxton CH, Leeds AR. Black Tea–Helpful or Harmful? A Review of the Evidence. *Eur J Clin Nutr.* 2007;61(1):3-18. doi:10.1038/sj.ejcn.1602489.

144. Chacko SM, Thambi PT, Kuttan R, Nishigaki I. Beneficial Effects of Green Tea: A Literature Review. *Chin Med.* 2010;5:13. doi:10.1186/1749-8546-5-13.

145. Mancini E, Beglinger C, Drewe J, Zanchi D. Green Tea Effects on Cognition, Mood, and Human Brain Function: A Systematic Review. *Phytomedicine.* 2017;34:26-37. doi:10.1016/j.phymed.2017.07.008.

146. Hodgson JM, Croft KD. Tea Flavonoids and Cardiovascular Health. *Mol Aspects Med.* 2010;31(6):495-502. doi:10.1016/j.mam.2010.09.004.

147. Huang J, Wang Y, Xie Z, Zhou Y, Zhang Y, Wan X. The Anti-Obesity Effects of Green Tea in Human Intervention and Basic Molecular Studies. *Eur J Clin Nutr.* 2014;68(10):1075-1087. doi:10.1038/ejcn.2014.143.

148. Fujiki H, Sueoka E, Watanabe T, Suganuma M. Primary Cancer Prevention by Green Tea, and Tertiary Cancer Prevention by the Combination of Green Tea Catechins and Anticancer Compounds. *J Cancer Res Clin Oncol.* 2012;138(8):1259-1270. doi:10.1007/s00432-012-1236-5.

149. Ros E. Health Benefits of Nut Consumption. *Nutrients.* 2010;2(7):652-682. doi:10.3390/nu2070652.

150. Wang X, Ouyang Y, Liu J, et al. Fruit and Vegetable Consumption and Mortality From All Causes, Cardiovascular Disease, and Cancer: Systematic Review and Dose-Response Meta-Analysis of Prospective Cohort Studies. *BMJ.* 2014;349:g4490. doi:10.1136/bmj.g4490.

151. Guasch-Ferré M, Liu X, Malik VS, et al. Nut Consumption and Risk of Cardiovascular Disease. *J Am Coll Cardiol.* 2017;70(20):2519-2532. doi:10.1016/j.jacc.2017.09.035.

152. Micha R, Peñalvo JL, Cudhea F, et al. Association Between Dietary Factors and Mortality From Heart Disease, Stroke, and Type 2 Diabetes in the United States. *JAMA.* 2017;317(9):912-924. doi:10.1001/jama.2017.0947.

References

153. Esfahani A, Wong JM, Truan J, et al. Health Effects of Mixed Fruit and Vegetable Concentrates: A Systematic Review of the Clinical Interventions. *J Am Coll Nutr.* 2011;30(5):285-294. doi:10.1080/07315724.2011.10719974.

154. Slavin JL. Fiber and Prebiotics: Mechanisms and Health Benefits. *Nutrients.* 2013;5(4):1417-1435. doi:10.3390/nu5041417.

155. National Institutes of Health (NIH). Nutrition and Health: Macronutrients and Micronutrients. Updated 2023. https://www.nih.gov/health-information/nutrition

156. World Health Organization (WHO). Healthy Diet Factsheet. Updated April 2023. https://www.who.int/news-room/fact-sheets/detail/healthy-diet

157. Harvard T.H. Chan School of Public Health. The Importance of Eating a Balanced Diet. Updated 2024. https://www.hsph.harvard.edu/nutritionsource/balanced-diet

158. Mayo Clinic. Nutrition Basics for Supporting Body Health. Published 2022. https://www.mayoclinic.org/nutrition

159. Academy of Nutrition and Dietetics. Building a Balanced Plate: Nutrient Needs for Health. Updated 2023. https://www.eatright.org/health

160. McArdle WD, Katch FI, Katch VL. Essentials of Exercise Physiology. 5th ed. Wolters Kluwer; 2019.

161. Guyton AC, Hall JE. Textbook of Medical Physiology. 13th ed. Elsevier; 2016.

162. National Institutes of Health (NIH). Understanding Body Composition. Updated 2023. https://www.nih.gov/

163. Centers for Disease Control and Prevention (CDC). Nutrition for Everyone: Macronutrients. Updated 2023. https://www.cdc.gov/nutrition/

164. World Health Organization (WHO). Carbohydrates and Human Nutrition. Updated 2022. https://www.who.int/news-room/fact-sheets/detail/carbohydrates-and-health

165. National Institutes of Health (NIH). Dietary Supplement Fact Sheets. Updated 2023. https://ods.od.nih.gov/factsheets/

166. U.S. Department of Agriculture (USDA). Macronutrients: Carbohydrates, Proteins, and Fats. Updated 2023. https://www.nutrition.gov/topics/whats-food/macronutrients

167. World Health Organization (WHO). Micronutrient Deficiencies. Updated 2023. https://www.who.int/health-topics/micronutrients

168. Harvard T.H. Chan School of Public Health. Phytochemicals: The Nutrition Powerhouse in Plants. Updated 2024. . https://www.hsph.harvard.edu/nutritionsource/antioxidants/

169. Centers for Disease Control and Prevention (CDC). Vitamins and Minerals. Updated 2023. https://www.cdc.gov/nutrition/resources-publications/vitamins-minerals.html

170. Mayo Clinic. Nutrition Basics: Macronutrients and Micronutrients. Published 2022. https://www.mayoclinic.org/nutrition-basics

171. Health effects of vegan diets. *The American Journal of Clinical Nutrition.* https://ajcn.nutrition.org/article/S0002-9165%2823%2923835-6/fulltext

172. Vegan nutrition. *Wikipedia.* https://en.wikipedia.org/wiki/Vegan_nutrition

173. Veganism. *Wikipedia.* https://en.wikipedia.org/wiki/Veganism

174. Evidence of a vegan diet for health benefits and risks – an umbrella review of meta-analyses of observational and clinical studies. *Critical Reviews in Food Science and Nutrition.* https://www.tandfonline.com/doi/pdf/10.1080/10408398.2022.2075311

175. Plant-based diet. *Wikipedia.* https://en.wikipedia.org/wiki/Plant-based_diet

176. Paoli A, Rubini A, Volek JS, Grimaldi KA. Beyond Weight Loss: A Review of the Therapeutic Uses of Very-Low-Carbohydrate (Ketogenic) Diets. *Eur J Clin Nutr.* 2013;67(8):789-796. doi:10.1038/ejcn.2013.116.

177. Fleming P, Godwin M. Low-Carbohydrate Diets in the Management of Obesity and Other Cardiometabolic Risk Factors: A Review of the Evidence. *Can Fam Physician.* 2013;59(7):653-655.

178. O'Keefe JH, Bell DSH. Postprandial Hyperglycemia/Hypoglycemia and Cardiovascular Disease: Cardio-Metabolic Risk and Dietary Strategies. *Mayo Clin Proc.* 2007;82(10):1221-1230. doi:10.4065/82.10.1221.

179. Whalen KA, Judd S, McCullough M, et al. Paleolithic and Mediterranean Diet Pattern Scores and Risk of Incident Colorectal Cancer. *Am J Epidemiol.* 2017;185(1):50-60. doi:10.1093/aje/kww224.

180. Estruch R, Ros E, Salas-Salvadó J, et al. Primary Prevention of Cardiovascular Disease with a Mediterranean Diet Supplemented with Extra-Virgin Olive Oil or Nuts. *N Engl J Med.* 2018;378(25):e34. doi:10.1056/NEJMoa1800389.

181. Baudry J, Touvier M, Allès B, et al. Association Between Organic Food Consumption and Cancer Risk: Findings From the NutriNet-Santé Prospective Cohort Study. *JAMA Intern Med.* 2018;178(12):1597-1606. doi:10.1001/jamainternmed.2018.4357.

182. Oxford University. Eating Organic Food Doesn't Lower Your Overall Risk of Cancer. Published March 28, 2014. https://www.ox.ac.uk/news/2014-03-28-eating-organic-food-doesnt-lower-your-overall-risk-cancer

183. Cornucopia Institute. New Study: Organic Diet Lowers Cancer Risk. Published October 2018. https://www.cornucopia.org/2018/10/new-study-organic-diet-lowers-cancer-risk/

184. Stanford Medicine. Little Evidence of Health Benefits from Organic Foods, Study Finds. Published September 2012. https://med.stanford.edu/news/all-news/2012/09/little-evidence-of-health-benefits-from-organic-foods-study-finds.html

185. European Journal of Environmental Health. Organic Food Consumption and Risk of Allergic Diseases and Obesity: A Systematic Review. *Environmental Health.* 2017;16:10. doi:10.1186/s12940-017-0315-4.

186. World Health Organization (WHO). Genetically Modified Organisms (GMOs): Frequently Asked Questions. Updated 2022. https://www.who.int/news-room/questions-and-answers/item/food-genetically-modified

187. GMO UCONN. GMOs and Human Health. Updated December 2023. https://gmo.uconn.edu/topics/gmos-and-human-health

188. Frontiers in Public Health. Pesticides and Human Health: A Review of Recent Studies. *Front Public Health.* 2016;4:148. doi:10.3389/fpubh.2016.00148.

189. Food and Wine. A New Study Reveals a Potential Link Between Pesticides and Prostate Cancer. Published September 2024. https://www.foodandwine.com/pesticides-prostate-cancer-risk-8739772

190. U.S. Food and Drug Administration. GMO Crops, Animal Food, and Beyond. https://www.fda.gov/food/agricultural-biotechnology/gmo-crops-animal-food-and-beyond

191. GMO Answers. GMO Crops On The Market in the U.S. https://gmoanswers.com/gmos-in-the-us

192. Center for Food Safety. About Genetically Engineered Foods. https://www.centerforfoodsafety.org/issues/311/ge-foods/about-ge-foods

193. HowStuffWorks. 10 Common Genetically Modified Foods. https://recipes.howstuffworks.com/5-common-genetically-modified-foods.htm

194. Environmental Working Group. PCBs in Farmed Salmon. https://www.ewg.org/research/pcbs-farmed-salmon

195. Center for Food Safety. Human Health Risks. https://www.centerforfoodsafety.org/issues/312/aquaculture/human-health-risks

196. Environmental Health News. Fish farming has a plastic problem. https://www.ehn.org/plastic-in-farmed-fish-2650268080.html

197. Center for Food Safety. Human Health Risks. https://www.centerforfoodsafety.org/issues/312/aquaculture/human-health-risks

198. Quadragroup. Seed Crushing: Enhancing Oil Extraction and Refinement. https://quadragroup.com/en-ca/insight-and-events/seed-crushing-enhancing-oil-extraction-and-refinement

199. Penn State Extension. Processing Edible Oils. https://extension.psu.edu/processing-edible-oils

200. Anderson International Corp. Understanding Hexane Extraction of Vegetable Oils. https://www.andersonintl.com/understanding-hexane-extraction-of-vegetable-oils/

201. Oklahoma State University Extension. Oil and Oilseed Processing II. https://extension.okstate.edu/fact-sheets/oil-and-oilseed-processing-ii.html

202. International Journal of Advanced Technology and Science Research. A Review on Health Risks from Processing Contaminants in Refined Edible Oils. https://www.ijatsr.org/assets/papers/2021/mar/ijatsr_02__12.pdf

203. Centers for Disease Control and Prevention. About Moderate Alcohol Use. https://www.cdc.gov/alcohol/about-alcohol-use/moderate-alcohol-use.html

204. World Health Organization. No Level of Alcohol Consumption is Safe for Our Health. https://www.who.int/europe/news-room/04-01-2023-no-level-of-alcohol-consumption-is-safe-for-our-health

205. Centers for Disease Control and Prevention. Alcohol Use and Your Health. https://www.cdc.gov/alcohol/about-alcohol-use/index.html

206. EatingWell. Even Moderate Drinking Might Be Too Much, U.S. Surgeon General Says —Here's Why. https://www.eatingwell.com/alcohol-cancer-warning-surgeon-general-8770746

207. Reuters. Explainer: How Alcohol Consumption Impacts Cancer Risk. https://www.reuters.com/business/healthcare-pharmaceuticals/how-alcohol-consumption-impacts-cancer-risk-2025-01-03/

208. Centers for Disease Control and Prevention. Alcohol and Public Health. https://www.cdc.gov/alcohol/index.htm

209. National Institutes of Health. What Are the U.S. Guidelines for Drinking? https://rethinkingdrinking.niaaa.nih.gov/how-much-is-too-much/what-are-the-us-guidelines-for-drinking.aspx

210. World Health Organization. Alcohol. https://www.who.int/news-room/fact-sheets/detail/alcohol

References

211. Centers for Disease Control and Prevention. Alcohol Use and Your Health. https://www.cdc.gov/alcohol/fact-sheets/alcohol-use.htm

212. National Institute on Alcohol Abuse and Alcoholism. Alcohol's Effects on the Body. https://www.niaaa.nih.gov/alcohols-effects-health/alcohols-effects-body

213. U.S. Food and Drug Administration (FDA). Food Additive Status List. Updated November 2022. https://www.fda.gov/food/food-additives-petitions/food-additive-status-list

214. Environmental Working Group (EWG). The Dirty Dozen and Clean Fifteen. Published 2023. https://www.ewg.org/foodnews/

215. National Cancer Institute. Artificial Sweeteners and Cancer Risk. Updated October 2023. https://www.cancer.gov/about-cancer/causes-prevention/risk/diet/artificial-sweeteners-fact-sheet

216. Center for Science in the Public Interest (CSPI). Chemical Cuisine: Additives to Avoid. Published 2022. https://www.cspinet.org/eating-healthy/chemical-cuisine

217. American Heart Association (AHA). Added Sugars. Published 2022. https://www.heart.org/en/healthy-living/healthy-eating/eat-smart/sugar

218. World Health Organization (WHO). Pesticide Residues in Food. Updated September 2022. https://www.who.int/news-room/fact-sheets/detail/pesticide-residues-in-food

219. International Federation for Produce Standards (IFPS). Price Look-Up (PLU) Codes. Published 2024. https://www.ifpsglobal.com/PLU-Codes

220. Turner-McGrievy GM, Wilcox S, Frongillo EA. The role of diet in inflammation: A review of potential mechanisms and evidence. *Am J Lifestyle Med.* 2019;13(4):e92-e105.

221. U.S. Department of Health and Human Services. Dietary Guidelines for Americans 2020-2025.

222. Zhang L, Rana I, Shaffer RM, Taioli E, Sheppard L. Exposure to glyphosate-based herbicides and risk for non-Hodgkin lymphoma: A meta-analysis and supporting evidence. *Mutat Res.* 2019;781:186-206. doi:10.1016/j.mrrev.2019.02.001

223. Koutros S, Silverman DT, Alavanja MC, et al. Occupational exposure to pesticides and prostate cancer risk in the Agricultural Health Study. *Int J Cancer.* 2013;132(2):377-384. doi:10.1002/ijc.27676

224. Bonner MR, Freeman LE, Hoppin JA, et al. Occupational exposure to chlorpyrifos and lung cancer incidence among pesticide applicators in the Agricultural Health Study. *Environ Health Perspect.* 2010;118(12):1766-1771. doi:10.1289/ehp.1002238

225. Chen M, Chang CH, Tao L, Lu C. Residential exposure to pesticide during childhood and childhood cancers: A meta-analysis. *Pediatrics.* 2015;136(4):719-729. doi:10.1542/peds.2015-0006

226. Aschebrook-Kilfoy B, Heltshe SL, Nuckols JR, et al. Modeled nitrate levels in well water supplies and prevalence of abnormal thyroid conditions among the agricultural health study cohort. *Occup Environ Med.* 2012;69(5):365-370. doi:10.1136/oemed-2011-100382

227. López-Carrillo L, Hernández-Ramírez RU, Gandolfi AJ, et al. Exposure to organochlorine pesticides and breast cancer: A meta-analysis. *Environ Health Perspect.* 2017;125(10):107002. doi:10.1289/EHP1308

References

228. Swallow DM. Genetics of lactase persistence and lactose intolerance. *Annu Rev Genet.* 2003;37:197-219. doi:10.1146/annurev.genet.37.110801.143820

229. Ingram CJ, Mulcare CA, Itan Y, Thomas MG, Swallow DM. Lactose digestion and the evolutionary genetics of lactase persistence. *Hum Genet.* 2009;124(6):579-591. doi:10.1007/s00439-008-0593-6

230. Tishkoff SA, Reed FA, Ranciaro A, et al. Convergent adaptation of human lactase persistence in Africa and Europe. *Nat Genet.* 2007;39(1):31-40. doi:10.1038/ng1946

231. Mattar R, de Campos Mazo DF, Carrilho FJ. Lactose intolerance: Diagnosis, genetic, and clinical factors. *Clin Exp Gastroenterol.* 2012;5:113-121. doi:10.2147/CEG.S32368

232. Shrier I, Szilagyi A, Rasko D, Seidman E. Lactose intolerance and its diagnosis: A review of genetic and clinical factors. *Pediatrics.* 2006;118(3):1279-1286. doi:10.1542/peds.2006-0508

233. Gerbault P, Moret C, Currat M, Sanchez-Mazas A. Impact of lactase persistence on human history. *Philos Trans R Soc B.* 2011;366(1566):863-877. doi:10.1098/rstb.2010.0268

234. JAMA Network Open. Association Between Ultra-Processed Food Consumption and Depression. Available from: https://jamanetwork.com/journals/jamanetworkopen/fullarticle/2809727

235. Harvard School of Public Health. Ultra-Processed Foods and Depression. Available from: https://hsph.harvard.edu/news/ultra-processed-foods-may-increase-risk-of-depression/

236. Frontiers in Nutrition. Neotame consumption and its impact on gut microbiota: A dysbiosis perspective. *Front Nutr.* 2024;11:1366409. doi:10.3389/fnut.2024.1366409.

237. Cedars-Sinai. Research Alert: Artificial sweeteners significantly alter the small bowel microbiome. *iScience.* 2024;28(3):100123. doi:10.1016/j.isci.2024.100123.

238. Suez J, Korem T, Zilberman-Schapira G, et al. Artificial sweeteners induce glucose intolerance by altering the gut microbiota. *Nat Med.* 2022;28(10):1343-1350. doi:10.1038/s41591-022-02063-z.

239. Fasano A, Catassi C. Clinical practice. Celiac disease. *N Engl J Med.* 2012;367(25):2419-2426. doi:10.1056/NEJMcp1113994

240. Lebwohl B, Sanders DS, Green PHR. Coeliac disease. *Lancet.* 2018;391(10115):70-81. doi:10.1016/S0140-6736(17)31796-8

241. Junker Y, Zeissig S, Kim S-M, et al. Wheat amylase trypsin inhibitors drive intestinal inflammation via activation of myeloid cells. *Gastroenterology.* 2012;143(4):1105-1115. doi:10.1053/j.gastro.2012.07.016

242. Biesiekierski JR, Newnham ED, Irving PM, et al. Gluten causes gastrointestinal symptoms in subjects without celiac disease: a double-blind randomized placebo-controlled trial. *Am J Gastroenterol.* 2011;106(3):508-514. doi:10.1038/ajg.2010.487

243. International Agency for Research on Cancer (IARC). IARC Monographs on the Evaluation of Carcinogenic Risks to Humans. Group 1 Carcinogens. Updated 2023. https://monographs.iarc.fr/list-of-classifications. Accessed [insert access date].

244. Journal of Food Protection. Aflatoxin contamination in peanuts: prevalence and safety measures. J Food Prot. 2015;78(7):1271-1281. doi:10.4315/0362-028X.JFP-14-332.

References

245. World Health Organization (WHO). Aflatoxins in food: exposure and health impacts. Updated October 2023. https://www.who.int/foodsafety/areas_work/chemical-risks/aflatoxins/en/. Accessed [insert access date].

246. European Food Safety Authority (EFSA). Maximum residue levels for aflatoxins in peanuts and related products.Published 2018. https://www.efsa.europa.eu/en/efsajournal/pub/5108. Accessed [insert access date].

247. International Agency for Research on Cancer (IARC). Acrylamide in food and cancer risk. Published 2015. https://www.iarc.fr. Accessed [insert access date].

248. World Health Organization (WHO). Frequently Asked Questions on Genetically Modified Foods. Updated 2022. https://www.who.int/foodsafety/areas_work/food-technology/faq-genetically-modified-food/en/. Accessed [insert access date].

249. U.S. Food and Drug Administration (FDA). GMO Crops, Animal Food, and Beyond. Updated December 2023. https://www.fda.gov/food/agricultural-biotechnology/gmo-crops-animal-food-and-beyond. Accessed [insert access date].

250. National Academies of Sciences, Engineering, and Medicine. Genetically Engineered Crops: Experiences and Prospects. National Academies Press; 2016. doi:10.17226/23395.

251. World Health Organization (WHO). Aflatoxins in food: exposure and health impacts. Updated October 2023. https://www.who.int/news-room/fact-sheets/detail/mycotoxins. Accessed [insert access date].

252. Kumar P, Mahato DK, Kamle M, Mohanta TK, Kang SG. Aflatoxins: a global concern for food safety, human health, and their management. *Front Microbiol*. 2017;7:2170. doi:10.3389/fmicb.2016.02170.

253. Wild CP, Gong YY. Mycotoxins and human disease: a largely ignored global health issue. *Carcinogenesis*.2010;31(1):71-82. doi:10.1093/carcin/bgp264.

254. Magan N, Aldred D. Post-harvest control strategies: minimizing mycotoxins in the food chain. *Int J Food Microbiol*. 2007;119(1-2):131-139. doi:10.1016/j.ijfoodmicro.2007.07.034.

255. Otsuki T, Wilson JS, Sewadeh M. What price precaution? European harmonization of aflatoxin regulations and African groundnut exports. *Eur Rev Agric Econ*. 2001;28(3):263-284. doi:10.1093/erae/28.3.263.

256. Williams JH, Phillips TD, Jolly PE, Stiles JK, Jolly CM, Aggarwal D. Human aflatoxicosis in developing countries: a review of toxicology, exposure, potential health consequences, and interventions. *Am J Clin Nutr*.2004;80(5):1106-1122. doi:10.1093/ajcn/80.5.1106.

257. Journal of Food Protection. Aflatoxin contamination in peanuts: prevalence and safety measures. *J Food Prot*.2015;78(7):1271-1281. doi:10.4315/0362-028X.JFP-14-332.

258. Kolok AS, Sellin MK. The environmental impact of growth-promoting compounds employed by the United States beef cattle industry: History, current knowledge, and future directions. *Environ Health Perspect*. 2020;128(8):085001. doi:10.1289/EHP4809

259. Suez J, Korem T, Zeevi D, et al. Artificial sweeteners induce glucose intolerance by altering the gut microbiota. *Nature*. 2014;514(7521):181-186. doi:10.1038/nature13793

References

260. International Agency for Research on Cancer (IARC). Styrene. In: *IARC Monographs on the Evaluation of Carcinogenic Risks to Humans.* Vol. 121. Lyon, France: World Health Organization; 2018.

261. Mann T, Tomiyama AJ, Westling E, Lew AM, Samuels B, Chatman J. Medicare's search for effective obesity treatments: diets are not the answer. *Am Psychol.* 2007;62(3):220-233.

262. Seidelmann SB, Claggett B, Cheng S, et al. Dietary carbohydrate intake and mortality: a prospective cohort study and meta-analysis. *Lancet Public Health.* 2018;3(9):e419-e428.

263. Budoff M, et al. Carbohydrate restriction-induced elevations in LDL-cholesterol and atherosclerosis: randomized controlled feeding trial. *JACC Adv.* 2024;3:101109.

264. Wang Z, Chen T, Wu S, et al. Impact of the ketogenic diet as a dietary approach on cardiovascular disease risk factors: a meta-analysis of randomized clinical trials. *Am J Clin Nutr.* 2024;120(3):e1-e12.

265. Gallop MR, et al. A long-term ketogenic diet causes hyperlipidemia, liver dysfunction, and glucose intolerance from impaired insulin secretion in mice. *Sci Adv.* 2025;11(38):eadx2752.

266. Noto H, Goto A, Tsujimoto T, Noda M. Low-carbohydrate diets and all-cause mortality: a systematic review and meta-analysis of observational studies. *PLoS One.* 2013;8(1):e55030.

267. Fu J, Bonder MJ, Cenit MC, et al. Dietary fiber intake and gut microbiota in human health. *Nutrients.* 2022;14(24):1-20.

268. Bouvard V, Loomis D, Guyton KZ, et al. Carcinogenicity of consumption of red and processed meat. *Lancet Oncol.* 2015;16(16):1599-1600.

269. International Agency for Research on Cancer. *Red Meat and Processed Meat.* IARC Monographs Volume 114. Lyon, France: IARC; 2018.

270. Pan A, Sun Q, Bernstein AM, et al. Red meat consumption and risk of type 2 diabetes: 3 cohorts of US adults and an updated meta-analysis. *Am J Clin Nutr.* 2011;94(4):1088-1096.

271. Manheimer EW, van Zuuren EJ, Fedorowicz Z, Pijl H. Paleolithic nutrition for metabolic syndrome: systematic review and meta-analysis. *Am J Clin Nutr.* 2015;102(4):922-932.

272. Genoni A, Christophersen CT, Lo J, et al. Long-term Paleolithic diet is associated with lower resistant starch intake, different gut microbiota composition, and increased serum TMAO concentrations. *Eur J Nutr.* 2020;59(5):1845-1858.

273. Pawlak R, Lester SE, Babatunde T. How prevalent is vitamin B12 deficiency among vegetarians? *Nutr Rev.* 2013;71(2):110-117.

274. Pawlak R, Parrott SJ, Raj S, Cullum-Dugan D, Lucus D. The prevalence of cobalamin deficiency among vegetarians assessed by serum vitamin B12: a review. *Eur J Clin Nutr.* 2014;68(5):541-548.

275. Tong TYN, Appleby PN, Bradbury KE, et al. Vegetarian and vegan diets and risks of total and site-specific fractures: results from the prospective EPIC-Oxford study. *BMC Med.* 2020;18:353.

276. Ballarin RS, et al. Vegetarian and vegan diets and the risk of hip fracture: systematic review and meta-analysis. *Nutr Rev.* 2025.

References

277. Filippou CD, Tsioufis CP, Thomopoulos CG, et al. Dietary Approaches to Stop Hypertension (DASH) diet and blood pressure reduction in adults with and without hypertension: a systematic review and meta-analysis of randomized controlled trials. *Adv Nutr.* 2020;11(5):1150-1160.
278. Klein AV, Kiat H. Detox diets for toxin elimination and weight management: a critical review of the evidence. *J Hum Nutr Diet.* 2015;28(6):675-686.
279. Sardaro MLS, et al. Effects of vegetable and fruit juicing on gut and oral microbiome composition: a dietary intervention study. *Nutrients.* 2025.
280. Northwestern University. Juicing may harm your health in just three days, study finds. 2025.
281. Pahlavani N, et al. The effects of a raw vegetarian diet from a clinical perspective: review of the available evidence. *Clin Nutr Open Sci.* 2023.

www.ingramcontent.com/pod-product-compliance
Lightning Source LLC
Chambersburg PA
CBHW040623030426
42322CB00061B/1997